NEVER

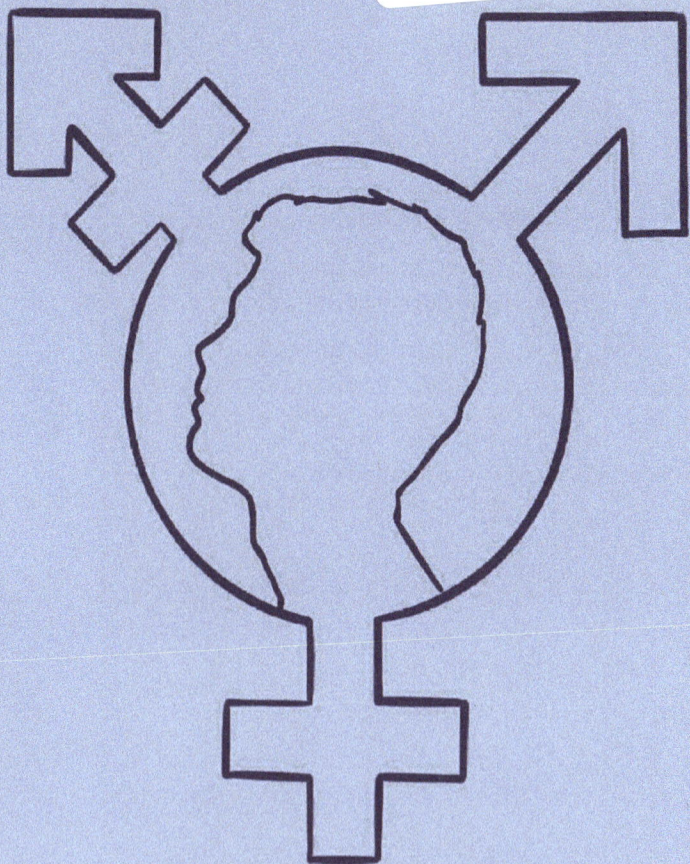

BY DANIEL KYE CANTER

This book is published by
Grosvenor House Publishing Ltd
Link House
140 The Broadway, Tolworth, Surrey, KT6 7HT.
www.grosvenorhousepublishing.co.uk

A CIP record for this book
is available from the British Library

ISBN 978-1-83975-611-5

IN MEMORY OF

My book is in memory of Carolyn Steele - a self-published author and also my cousin.

When I began to write my story, I sent some tentative first chapters to her so that she could give them the 'once-over'. She, very meticulously, read my scribblings and made some notes on how I could add more detail and more feeling to my writing.

Her knowledge and wisdom helped me to express myself more clearly and I can't thank her enough for her input.

Very sadly, Carolyn has since passed away, but I know she would have been proud to read my story, and I am so sad that she didn't get the chance.

DEDICATIONS

There are three people to whom I would like to dedicate this book:

The first person is my friend Sam who passed away before I finished my physical transition. The last time we met, I had only had chest surgery and was waiting for my first genital surgery.

Sam was so excited that I had decided to fully transition from female to male as he knew how happy I was becoming even at the very beginning of the process, and he would have wanted to see me fulfil my dream of becoming the man I should have always have been.

So, Sam, if Kindle is available wherever you are, please feel free to download a copy!

The second person to whom I would like to dedicate this book is Karen Without her patience, selflessness and understanding, I am not sure I would be where I am now. She gave me the gentle nudges I needed to explore my deepest feelings without a thought for her own potential losses. I am, and always will be, so grateful to her. Our ongoing friendship is testament to her accepting nature, and I thank her for being there for me when I needed her.

The third person is my beautiful wife Carla, without whom I am not sure I would have coped. She is not only my friend, my soulmate, and my wife and lover, she was also my nurse and my emotional rock throughout my transition. I thank her for her unwavering care, love and support. She has always held out a strong hand for me to squeeze as tightly as I needed through the good times and the bad, and I would have been so lost without her.

THANKS AND ACKNOWLEDGEMENTS

I would like to thank my friend Tyler Kennett, fondly known as 'my little brother from another mother', for the artwork he produced for my book, as shown on the front cover, the title page, the back cover and on 'Trans' umbrella diagram.

Tyler agreed to do this for me at a time when he was inundated with art coursework and, for that, I am truly grateful!

He is an amazing and inspirational young artist and, not only am I thankful to have him as a friend, I am also so honoured to be able to include some of his work in my book.

You can find him on his social media platforms, as below:

Facebook – Tyler Kennett Art
Instagram – @tylerkennettart

I want to say a massive thank to my Mum for offering to proof-read my book for me over five years ago when I first began writing. I actually wrote half of this book and then stopped for many reasons - surgeries, work and life, to name just a few. I wasn't actually sure I would ever finish it, but after some encouragement from Mum and having been given some impromptu time off work due to Covid-19, I was able to pour some much-needed time and effort into finishing it.

I sent my manuscript to Mum in an email and didn't expect her to hand it back for many months. But she worked on it every day and made sure that my grammar and punctuation were correct and that the sentences flowed nicely. Her attention to detail is amazing and we both wanted to make sure that when I sent it for editing, it would be the best version that it could be. We both knew that an editor would make changes, but we still wanted it to be right beforehand.

I also want to thank Mum for her acceptance and non-judgemental attitude toward me throughout my life. I have been through many different stages before finally realising what I needed to do and who I needed to be, and she would always just support me and help me through each of these stages.

Mum is not shy and would always tell me her opinion even if I didn't want to hear it. She would never try to change me or my opinions or choices, but she would try to show different sides to a situation. I now realise that this was, and always will be, born of love, even if I didn't realise it at the time.

I want to also thank my Dad for being such a laid-back 'dude', taking everything in his stride. He never questioned my thought processes or judgements; he just supported and did what he could to make things as easy for me as was possible.

I would also like to extend my gratitude to my wider family and friends. They have all been amazing and have shown nothing but true acceptance. My choices were never questioned and for that I am, and will always be, truly grateful.

There is one friend in particular that I will just call A. I would like to thank her for those times we shared together on individual journeys, albeit in different directions. We shared so many commonalities, one being our humour and I think we both needed this at that particular time in our lives.

Introduction

My name is Daniel. I am a 46-year-old Transgender man, and I began my transition from female to male when I was 37 years old.

I came into the world in 1974 and was named Nikki.

My beautiful family

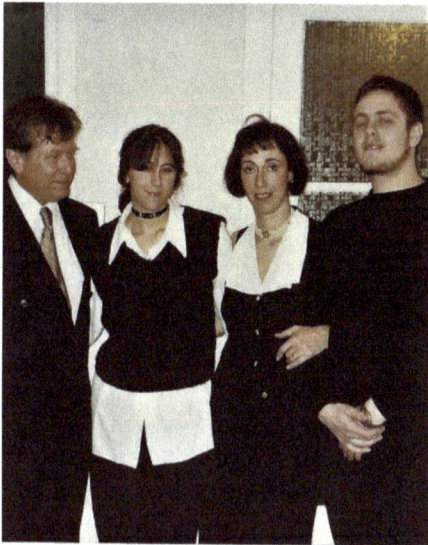

The picture below is one that was taken of me pre-transition and I wanted this to be used as a comparison photo to those at the end of the book, to show all the changes of medical and surgical transition.

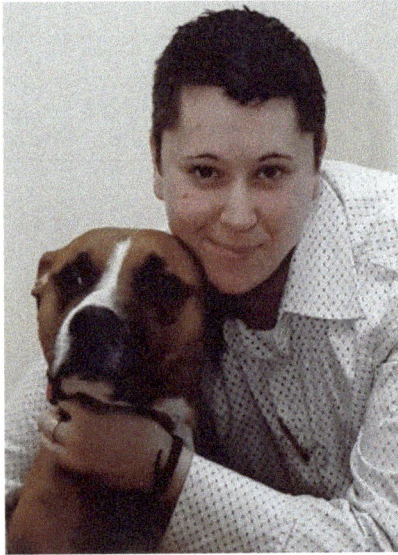

This is my story.
It is a frank, honest and open account of my life.

Warning:
There will be discussion of body parts and sexual experiences, including graphic post-surgery and naked images.

I was asked to write an article by Kay West, the President of the Beaumont Society with whom I had made contact early in my personal journey of discovery. My intention was to join the Society's support group, as I needed a place where

I could explore my thoughts around my gender, and the feelings that I was 'born in the wrong body' or was 'born in the wrong box'; this was how a dear friend described me after me telling her I was going to transition from female to male.

I spoke to the Director about the possibility of me joining the Society and I was welcomed with open arms. However, I was told that the Society was comprised, predominantly, of people who identified as female, but were born into a male body. She went on to tell me that she would really love to see the group expand to incorporate people who identified as male, but who were born into a female body. It was not that the group was not inclusive, it was just that the Society seemed to attract the former group of people.

The idea behind the article was that I would introduce myself and tell my story over a series of quarterly magazine articles. The intention was to show the 'other side of the coin' and help other Transgender men to be able to access the support that the group offered.

The Society is a lifeline for so many in that it provides free and confidential support to people identifying as different from their birth gender. However, I would like to point out that I have learned that not everyone who is struggling with their identity wants to, nor feels the need to, transition medically or surgically. There are many forms of gender expression and there is so much diversity in the world.

Can you imagine the worry, turmoil and self-hatred that someone may feel, as they start to realise that their body does not match how they feel and wish to be seen, with the additional impact that this revelation will have on the lives of their loved-ones? This is a crucial time in a person's transition, and this is the time that they will really need to be supported and accepted.

Perhaps you might imagine a scenario where you have been happily married for twenty-five years and have two children. One evening, your husband tells you that he wants, and needs, to be a woman and that he wants to go through the process of transitioning from male to female. He cries when he tells you because of the dramatic relief he feels at getting this out into the open, yet he is petrified of what this will mean and how it could affect his marriage, his kids and, actually, his whole life. He has already prepared himself for the worst possible scenario, but even the thought of that is not enough to stop him telling his wife. Can you imagine how terrified you might be? How would you even begin a conversation like this one? What would be going through your head? I ask you these questions because I feel that it is really important to try to understand what someone may go through and that, perhaps, this insight may help.

Support groups are absolutely invaluable and essential, not only for the people who are going on their own journeys of discovery but, also, for their loved ones. What I have learned from my own transition is that it is not just about the individual, it is about their partners, their husbands, their wives, their children, their parents and friends, and so many more!

The journey that a person undertakes to become their true self can, at times, be long, arduous, scary and isolating and there is a real need for understanding, empathy and education.

The articles I wrote for the Beaumont Society were published, and were very well received, and that was the reason that I decided to write my story. I would like to take this opportunity to thank the Society for its support and for enabling me to help others on their own personal journeys.

I feel extremely proud and excited to tell my story. My hope in writing this book is that I may help people understand better, the needs and desires of someone who feels they are trapped in the wrong body. Not only that, I would like to show a broader picture and how this may impact the lives of those around us.

My aim is also to provide emotional, educational and supporting tools for anyone who may be going through transition or is thinking about it. I hope to give some perspective and guidance on what they may go through if they choose this pathway.

If I can accomplish any of these things, I will be a very happy man.

Chapter One - Misfit

Let's begin with a little background.

I had a happy early childhood but memories of this are very limited. However, I do remember being part of a functional family, full of love and adoration.

I think it is important to mention that some people think Gender Dysphoria (the condition of feeling one's emotional and psychological identity as male or female to be opposite to one's biological sex) stems from childhood trauma and feelings of being unloved. This was not the case for me; as I have already mentioned, my childhood was a happy one. However, this may be the case for some people but, as I'm not a psychologist, I will leave that to professionals to determine.

When I was younger, my parents chose what I would wear but, as I started to grow up, I chose my own clothes and seemed to naturally adopt a tomboy look. Mum and Dad never questioned my choices, they just let me express myself as I wished.

Within our society, it is generally much more acceptable for a girl to dress in boys' clothes, than it is the other way around. Imagine the anxieties experienced by boys who wished to dress in a more feminine way, not being able to express themselves and be true to the way they instinctively feel?

It was always very easy for me to dress in a boyish way without bringing any unwanted attention. At that time, I had no idea why I wanted to dress in male-style clothes; I just knew that I felt more comfortable dressing this way.

I reached puberty at around 12 years old and, although I wasn't really prepared for what was to come, it didn't really have a massive effect on me. I remember being on holiday with Mum and Dad and whilst there, I started having periods. I knew what they were and what they meant, but I didn't truly know what to expect. I didn't know that I was different to any other girl, other than thinking that I was a tomboy; I thought I was experiencing what every other girl experienced at that age. I started to develop breasts but, again, this didn't really bother me, I just accepted it all as part of growing up.

I always hated the academic part of my school life, but I was naturally gifted when it came to playing sport and this gave me a real focus. It also gave me a great excuse to wear more androgynous (partly male, partly female) clothing.

I had a very close circle of friends and, for the most part, these were happy days. During my time at secondary school, I began my first relationship with a girl. I can't say that I had ever considered being in a same-sex relationship, but it just seemed to evolve from a close friendship into a full-on relationship. We never discussed the fact that we wouldn't tell anyone that we were together, we just didn't. We spent a lot of time together as she was also into sport, and we developed a really close bond. Even though we didn't tell anyone, I was very sure that friends and family had worked it out for themselves. She ended the relationship after a year or so. She was my first love, and I was heartbroken.

Throughout my school life, I felt a strong desire to fit in and conform to the 'norm' and ended up having a string of meaningless relationships with boys and men. I also went through this period of time, dressing in a very feminine way – probably another way of conforming. I didn't like dressing like this, but I did it anyway.

After leaving school, I went on to complete a BTEC National Diploma in Leisure Studies with the intention of becoming a sports coach/teacher. I enjoyed my first year at college, but really struggled in the second year. I already felt a little distant from my peers, as they all seemed to have 'normal' lives and I just didn't feel I fitted in, but didn't know why at the time.

During the first year, I was due to go on a trip with the rest of my class-mates, but ended up missing it because I developed a throat infection. Because the rest of the class had really bonded on that trip, I felt a little 'out on a limb'. Also, by the second year, I had decided that I didn't want to pursue a career in sport, so this all made the second year quite awkward for me and I remember considering whether I should quit the course. I didn't, and managed to continue to the end and received a Distinction as my final grade.

After my BTEC had finished, I found a job in a pet shop as I loved animals and that was something that I knew I could do happily, but after having been there for a year or so, I started to experience some health issues.

After many visits to my GP, I was eventually referred to a specialist in the diagnosis and treatment of Myalgic Encephalomyelitis (ME for short). When I attended my appointment, I was, very quickly, diagnosed with ME, then sometimes known as 'yuppie flu', as all the symptoms I experienced were a good comparison with those associated with ME. Those symptoms were nausea, lethargy and feelings of depression and anxiety; there were others that were documented, but these are the only ones I experienced.

I took a year off work to try to recover but the depression quickly accelerated. I was at home all day and felt a useless waste of space. I didn't know what direction my life would take and I was bitterly unhappy.

Looking back, I wonder if some of those symptoms were related to Gender Dysphoria. I am not saying that I didn't have ME, but I can now see some links, especially to depression.

I met a guy a while later, and he seemed to be the answer to my prayers; handsome, friendly and intelligent. He was supportive about my health issues, but he was so involved with his studies, we ended up becoming distant. Things did improve once he had completed some of his work-load and, because we loved each other, I asked him to marry me.

As time went on, it became very apparent that he wanted children. I definitely did not want children and had zero maternal instinct. I would often question myself as to why I didn't want children? Surely that was a natural instinct for every woman?

Fortunately, we never married, as his desire to have children brought an end to our engagement. We managed to remain friends after having some time apart and, ironically, later on we came out to each other as gay.

I was still away from work and on a slippery slope to losing my identity, well, the identity I knew about. I had a fraught relationship with my Mum and I think that was because she had always been a bubbly and outgoing person and, because I was feeling so low, her character overwhelmed me and made me disappear into my shell even more. She tried so hard to help me get through my rough patch and to keep my spirits up and jolly me along, but I just felt that she didn't understand and I felt resentful toward her. I did question how could she possibly understand when I didn't understand myself? All I knew was that I felt low, depressed, lost and, now I think of it, angry.

The relationship I had with my Dad was a totally different one. He had always been a quiet, laid-back, unassuming man, so there were never really any challenges from him. I am not saying that Mum challenged me negatively, as I now realise that those challenges were born of love and affection.

I plodded along for a while but, finally, I decided I wanted to 'come out' to my friends and family and tell them that I was gay. I had just chosen to try to do the 'normal thing' for a while, but I knew that I was happiest when I was in that first relationship with a girl. When I told my friends and family, they were extremely supportive and told me that they had already guessed. I was so glad that they already knew as it made coming out to them so much easier. Now, I would be free to dress the way I really wanted to and I went back my tomboy style.

When I decided to return to work, I found a job at a sports shop and met a girl that I really liked. We worked together on most shifts and developed a close friendship, which then led us into a relationship. She was not openly gay, which caused me frustration because I was now 'out and proud'. We would argue constantly about why she was not willing to come out to friends and family. I now realise that she had made a choice that was right for her at that time and I now accept that she just didn't want to be 'out'. It was inevitable that the relationship would not stand the test of time, however, I was really upset when she ended it so abruptly.

I continued to have relationships with women and I tended to take on a 'butch' role. I fancied feminine girls, but actually ended up with some quite butch ones?! Nothing made sense!

In addition to my relationship confusion, I started to experience feelings about my body that I couldn't explain. Although I was by no means disgusted by my body, when I looked in the mirror, I really didn't like what I saw, as it didn't really fit with how I felt inside. I knew that I liked to dress in a masculine way and that I liked women more than men, but I had really no idea what that meant to me. Was I just gay and choosing to express myself in a more masculine way or was there more to it? Were these feelings 'normal' - I didn't think so? I felt so overwhelmed, and very unsure why I was feeling this way.

For as long as I can remember, I have wanted to stand and pee like a man; I did not want sit like a girl. This was such a strong feeling that, one day, whilst my parents were not around, I sneaked into the shed and found a funnel. I did this because I needed to see and feel what it would be like to stand and pee. When I tried it and it was amazing to see, but I didn't experience the actual feelings I wanted because, let's face it, I was peeing into a plastic funnel.

I also wanted to be able to walk around without wearing a top; I had feelings of envy toward boys/men, as they were, naturally, able to do what I wanted to do. They also looked the way I wanted to look and this seemed so unfair! I now realise that these feelings were more than just envy. I know plenty of women who have told me that they really wished they could stand and pee and bring an end to stinging their nether regions in fields whilst camping or at a festival. Also, I have been told that some wished they could walk around when the weather was hot without wearing anything on top. But there was a huge difference to what they wanted and how this was affecting me mentally.

I didn't know why I was feeling like this and I couldn't begin to imagine talking about it. I didn't actually tell anyone, not for quite some time anyway. When I did tell a partner, it was after we had split up as I was scared of her reaction. Even when I told her, I didn't really know what I was feeling and how significant it would become for my future.

As my breasts grew bigger, I began to dislike how they looked; I wanted a flat chest with nicely contoured pectoral muscles. My body just didn't look nor feel right to me. When I looked in the mirror and saw my reflection, it didn't match how I felt inside. I would often stand in front of the mirror for a while, visualising what I would look like with no breasts, and wondering if there was any surgery I could have to remove them. I really didn't know what that would involve, or if it could be done. Was there such a thing as changing your body? I felt embarrassed and ashamed of myself, so much so that I didn't even want to research it on the Internet.

I got into another gay relationship and we lived together for around two years. It was mostly a happy time, but I still had those feelings. I remember questioning myself constantly and thinking that I was a freak, not normal. As time went on, those feelings began to embed themselves more deeply, until it came to a point where it all became too much for me and I ended the relationship under a dark cloud of confusion and frustration.

Some time passed and I met another woman and we were together for a total of five years, a record in my book. During those five years, we went through a Civil Partnership ceremony and, finally, there was a commitment to be in a relationship for the long haul. But after just eighteen months of marriage, things changed. She broke off the relationship and filed for a dissolution of our Civil Partnership. I have chosen not to go into further detail about this as I don't want to tarnish her character by divulging the details.

Yet again, another failed relationship! What was so wrong with me, why didn't anything ever work out? My thoughts would often take me back to how I felt about my body. I wonder now, if she had picked up on anything from me without it being said? I didn't fight her on the decision to dissolve the Civil Partnership and now I wonder if this was because I thought that the dissolution was a good idea and, maybe, a saving grace, a 'get-out clause'. I moved back home for a period of time after that ended, as I needed to get my head straight.

Having moved back home, I began to notice that my being there was having a positive effect on my relationship with Mum. I was finally able to speak to her about the depression I went through due to the ME, and she told me that she had also gone through a rough patch some time earlier, as she had been depressed after some surgery. She elaborated by telling me that her depression was due to the confinement she felt after that surgery. Mum had always been a social butterfly and was always busy with friends, family, work and hobbies. The recovery from surgery was long and intense and she said that she felt isolated and that had an impact on her mental health.

She told me that what had also badly affected her was the relationship I was in at the time with the girl who was not 'out'. Mum said that she didn't like her as she was rude, unfriendly and definitely not right for me. These sentiments were also echoed by Dad, so Mum was not alone in thinking these things.

I was totally oblivious to how they felt and I suppose they didn't want to upset me or 'rock the boat' at the time by telling me. When she disclosed this, I realised what a detrimental impact this had had on Mum at that time and I felt ashamed that I had a part to play in her depression.

This was definitely a turning point for Mum and me. She admitted that she knew how awful I must have been feeling when I was going through my rough patch and we found some common ground. This was a new and different relationship to the one that we had before. We had reached a better understanding of each other and a new appreciation of what the other had been through. Don't get me wrong, I always loved my Mum and I know that she definitely loved me and nothing changed for us in that respect. I just think that her vivacious character overwhelmed me at times, especially when I was feeling so low. I felt very much in the shadows, not because she put me there, but because I was lost in my own feelings.

A while later, I moved out of London and away from everything and everyone I knew, to begin a new life in Kent with a new girlfriend. We rented a house together for a while, but guess what - this relationship didn't work out either. Feelings of failure, unhappiness and uselessness were rife in my head! I was well aware of my feelings, but my partners were not and this had a huge effect on everyone around me, especially my partners. They gave me everything that I should have needed to feel happy, content and complete. I felt that there was a pattern developing, but I didn't know how to break the chain.

Despite the renewed understanding with my family, I still felt alone. I would quickly move to find someone else as I had such a strong urge to find happiness and companionship. I never gave myself the time to be alone with my feelings and just be at one with myself, jumping from one relationship to the next. I know now that this was not fair on my partners or me. If I didn't know who I was, how could anyone else be expected to understand me or know me?

I followed my usual pattern of searching for companionship and met another woman. She was a very supportive, understanding and positive woman. I finally felt as though I had fallen on my feet and felt comfortable enough to tell her my innermost secret. It was one night, whilst enjoying sitting in a hot tub together under the stars, that I started to tell her about how I was feeling. Her reaction was one of shock and surprise but that quickly turned into support and encouragement. I can't imagine what was going through her head when I told her. As far as she knew, she was in a relationship with a woman and here I was telling her that I felt like my body was wrong for me. At this point, I still couldn't really articulate my feelings very well because I still didn't understand them myself, but she just allowed me to talk and say what was in my head.

She was very interested and asked a lot of questions; she also tried to help me to think about things more clearly and to give those thoughts some sort of perspective. She said that she would be happy to help me explore my feelings and suggested that we go to gay bars together, where it would be safe for me to explore. She suggested that maybe I could dress in a more masculine way and see how it made me feel. For some reason, I chose not to take her up on her suggestion; maybe I wasn't yet ready for that.

When I told her how I felt, I was ready for her to be shocked and angry, but I wasn't ready for her to be so encouraging and supportive. This threw me a little as I had almost prepared for the worst. I was so grateful that she had reacted the way she had, as it gave me hope, and I felt excited that I may finally be able to be more the person that I felt I should be. However, I felt guilty because she was just so kind and understanding and I didn't really know how to deal with that guilt.

After some time, and having talked more about my feelings, she encouraged me to seek professional help. She believed that there were some deep underlying issues that needed to be explored. I agreed, as I knew that this was something that I should have done a long time ago.

Sadly, things became quite bad for us, to the point of almost splitting up. I knew that I had to do something about this or I was going to lose her and the life we had built together. I needed to deal with my issues and my problems with long-term commitment. We took a relationship break as we both needed time and space away from each other to be able to think more rationally. It was during this time apart, that I decided I should try to seek the help I needed to move on with my life. We re-ignited our relationship and things seemed better.

I asked her to marry me as we seemed to have rekindled our loving relationship and things were going really well for us. I truly believed that I was ready for that huge commitment all over again. With hindsight, I think I was just desperately searching for my 'happy ever after', and if I were going to be with anyone, it would have been her.

Unfortunately, as time went on, I started to become insular, non-communicative, selfish, reactive, and I felt pressured to show love and affection to her, when that should have come naturally to me I began to lose touch with reality and felt like I was spiralling downwards; it was horrible. I didn't understand my feelings, but I still chose to ignore them by hiding my head in the sand or up my own arse, for want of a better phrase. I was going to lose her.

I also started to lose touch with some of the friends from my past, but I tried desperately to keep hold of a few true friends from London, but even that became a struggle. However, I think this was my fault and, looking back, I think that it was probably me shutting down my past, trying to protect myself. I had, however, been introduced to some people by my partner and I had started to build some new friendships with a few people in Kent - new life, new friends.

Chapter Two - Out of the Shadows

I was now coming to a point where I knew I had to change things or I would lose everything and everyone that meant so much to me. I made a plan of all the things I would need to do to try to break this circle of failure.

MY PLAN:

<u>Phase One:</u>

I needed to have a frank and honest conversation with Mum and Dad. I had not even considered how or when this would take place, I just knew that it needed to happen before I could move on to the next phase.

I remember very clearly that my partner and I had gone to visit Mum and Dad for lunch one day and that we all sat outside on a lovely sunny day. I didn't realise then that I was going to have 'the conversation', as it hadn't yet entered my head. It was whilst helping Mum in the kitchen with the washing up that it all just 'came out'! I started by saying "I have something important to tell you". I told her how I felt that I had been born in the wrong body and how this had affected me in almost every area of my life. As always, Mum listened very intently before speaking but, when she did, she simply said "I know, I have always known". She told me that she would never have asked me about it because she wanted it to come from me. She also said, "nothing will change other than I gave birth to a son and a daughter, but now I have two sons".

She told me that she was extremely worried about me going through any kind of transition, as she knew that it would involve complicated and painful surgery. She actually knew more about transition, and what it involved, than I did. I knew that what she was saying came from a place of love and not because she disagreed with my decision.

When I talked to her, I felt emotional, but validated. There was no judgement and no selfishness from her. I mention selfishness because I have heard so many people say that, when they told their parents, the reaction they got was all about them, the parents. Some of the things that have been said are "what about me and how this is going to affect me" or "I feel like I'm going to lose the daughter/son I gave birth to". I cannot imagine how I would have felt if this had been the reaction I had received. I feel that this is extremely cruel and unsupportive as surely they would only care about their child. I have never understood this way of thinking because, to me, the person will remain the same person, they will just be changing their outer shell.

Mum asked me whether I wanted to tell my Dad, or if I would prefer her to do it. I said I would really appreciate her doing that, as it took some of the pressure off of me.

Again, other than concern for my emotional and physical well-being, there was nothing but acceptance and love from both of them. My Dad said to me "Why did you make me wait this long to get another Son?" I was truly overwhelmed by their love and acceptance of me.

Phase Two:

I planned a visit to my General Practitioner, with a view to a possible counselling referral and/or some antidepressants.

I needed some help to deal with the daily mental struggles about my body and my confidence, and the feeling that I was good for nothing; I was also trying to cope with a job which I disliked.

I made an appointment with my GP surgery for which I had to wait a couple of weeks, and I hoped that I would be seeing someone that I had seen before. When I attended the appointment, the GP I saw was a locum. I had not met him before, but he listened to me and showed empathy. He asked me to complete a brief questionnaire which was designed to show whether I was depressed and, if I was, how badly. Once he had ascertained that I was not suicidal, he diagnosed moderate depression and gave me a prescription for antidepressants, and also referred me to a psychiatrist.

Phase Three:

Referral to a psychiatrist. This was quite a scary prospect for me, as it meant revealing my innermost thoughts, feelings and desires, and it was something that I had never done before in such depth. It involved a lengthy consultation, culminating in a diagnosis of anxiety-related depression, but not psychiatric problems. I was certainly relieved to find out that I was not going mad and that my feelings were valid and just needed an outlet, which would be best achieved by consulting a psychologist.

Phase Four:

Referral to a psychologist for CBT (Cognitive Behavioural Therapy).I had four sessions which were covered by my private healthcare insurance. Following these sessions, I felt stronger, more confident and ready to further explore the deeper issue around my identity.

I found CBT to be really helpful and constructive, and the support given by the psychologist was the key to me acknowledging that I had gender-identity-related issues. She told me that I was not alone and that there were many people who felt as I did. This was a revelation to me and I began to feel less alone. She told me about the term 'Transgender' and what it meant, and she said that there was a possibility that many of my feelings were in line with the feelings that would be experienced by someone who was Transgender.

She armed me with the tools necessary to acknowledge, and deal with, my confidence issues. My homework was to research some support groups for Transgender (Trans) people. I was also asked to revisit my regular GP for a referral to the Gender Identity Clinic (GIC). I was stunned to learn that there was actually a clinic for people like me. It meant that I was definitely not alone. I remember feeling nervous, but also excited.

Phase Five:

Appointment with GP for referral to the GIC. I made an appointment to go back to my GP to discuss further, the possibility of being referred to the GIC. I had already begun to research what it meant to be Trans and what was involved in transitioning from female to male; I also wanted to find out about the help that would be accessible to me. I did some research on the GIC, the organisation where I would need to be referred. I wanted to gather as much information as I could before seeing my GP, to prove to him that I was serious about this and needed his help.

While researching information about the surgeries and what was involved in the transition process, I remember feeling shocked and extremely concerned about the cost implications. I had read that the total cost (if there were no complications requiring additional surgeries) could run to over £30,000. I knew that there would be no way that I could possibly fund this myself!

I began to look on online, to try to find out if transition costs were funded by the NHS and discovered that it was, as the medical processes and surgeries involved are not considered to be cosmetic. I was so relieved!

I was beginning to realise that transition was a very real prospect for me. I wanted this poignant time in my life to remain forever in my thoughts. After giving it some thought, I decided that a great way to begin the process would be to have a tattoo on my arm, so that I would see it every single day. I spent a long time looking at designs and deciding on the inscription. I knew that I wanted something personal, the meaning of which only I and a few others would understand. I chose an inscription in Latin- 'E Tenebris In Lucem' which translates as 'Out of the shadows and into the light'. I found a tattooist who could fit me in quite quickly and had it done. This is one tattoo, I know, I will never regret.

I was becoming curious about whether I could find a site on the Internet that sold some kind of fake willy or even a willy that I could actually use to pee through - did such a thing exist? I didn't need to look for long because when I typed in 'prosthetic penis to urinate through' so many sites came up. I chose a site based in Singapore because I liked the name of the company- Peecock Products^{TM}. This company manufactures and sells products for female to male, pre-op transgender people. I was so excited by what I saw on their website; it felt as if I were in a toy shop. I was shocked, but intrigued and inquisitive, when I saw all of the different types of products that were available.

These products were expensive, but after checking on some other sites, I decided that I liked the Peecock products and ended up choosing a willy that cost approximately 200 US Dollars. Although expensive, this was going to be an investment in my happiness and I hoped that it would be worth every penny.

Whilst exploring the site, I also discovered that they sold vests (called binders) that help to flatten the chest. I had no idea that these existed either, but was so happy to find that they did. I bought one which cost approximately 30 US Dollars. I couldn't wait to receive my package (pardon the pun) and sincerely hoped that there would be no company identity on the packaging - how embarrassing would that have been!

It only took about two and a half weeks to arrive and, thankfully, when it did, it was labelled very discreetly. I was so excited and I couldn't wait to get it open. I ripped through the packaging as though I knew there was gold inside. I quickly skimmed through the instructions and put it on. WOW - what a difference a bit of silicone can make! I put it on the way I thought it should be worn, but I discovered, to my horror, that it had begun to fall out of my pants. I made a small adjustment, followed by a lengthy pose in front of a full-length mirror, and then came a little cat-walk strutting, followed by further pauses in front of the mirror. You should have seen this; I was strutting around like a peacock that was trying to entice a female! I am sure it would have been absolutely hilarious to anyone watching.

The willy I had chosen was not the largest on the website. It was medium-sized, but most men would be proud to have one that size. I purposely didn't go for the large size because I was conscious that I would be wearing this thing in my everyday life. I didn't want to draw any unnecessary attention to myself, especially as this was all so new to me. I was happy with the size, and the appearance and, also, that it created a nice bulge in the right place.

Next on the agenda was to find out if, as the company claimed on their website, I could actually pee through this thing and set about drinking some fluids to aid me in my quest. In my excited state, I quickly realised that I hadn't read the instructions thoroughly enough and, inevitably, was a little overzealous and I leaked! When I say leaked, what I actually mean is that there was a nice steady stream of warm pee running down my legs and pooling on the floor at my feet- whoops! I re-read the instructions much more carefully this time, to make sure I wasn't wearing it in the wrong position, but it was okay, I just needed to control the flow. The instructions also suggested that I practice in the shower as this is safer. After drinking some more fluid, I gave it another try, this time in the shower. It was considerably harder to control the flow than I had realised but, this time, I was a little more successful. Several pees later, I had almost mastered the procedure, however, if I were bursting to go, then it could present more of a challenge.

There was also another, very important, feature of this willy; it would enable penetrative sex. In order to use it for this purpose, the company provided a rigid rod which had to be inserted into the hollow centre; this thing was amazing and I couldn't wait to try it all.

The idea was to wear this all the time, but I was worried about how people might react. Would anyone notice the bulge in my trousers? I began by wearing it whilst at home, so that I could get used to it and how it made me feel. I also wanted to make sure that I got the positioning right.

Once I felt more comfortable, I started to wear the prosthetic willy every day at work as well as at home. When I had, initially, looked at the website, I had seen that they sold harnesses that help the willy stay in the right place. I didn't buy one at that time, but now that I was wearing it at work, I thought that it would be a good plan to buy one. I had horrible thoughts of being at work and it slipping out of my pants and falling onto the floor. I could only imagine the horror of a work colleague walking up behind me saying "I think you dropped something". Although that scenario sounds utterly hilarious to me now, at the time I would have been mortified!

Wearing the prosthetic became a normal part of my daily life, and part of getting dressed in the morning. Although it was not part of my body, it was an extension of it and was the closest thing I could have that would make me feel more masculine.

At home, I began to notice my partner's reaction to me wearing it; she looked worried. This concerned me because I knew, just by looking at her face, that she didn't like what it represented. She had always identified as a lesbian and had never been with a male partner, so seeing this thing attached to me must have been completely alien to her. When we began our relationship, I was a woman and seeing me take these first steps towards the masculinisation of my body must have been really hard for her.

I wanted to talk to her about it, but I just didn't feel able to because, in my heart, I knew it could lead to a conversation about a possible break-up. She did, however, talk to me about it and told me how it made her feel when she saw me wearing it. She said that she was struggling with the reality of what it represented and what it would mean for us. I tried my hardest to understand, but it was difficult for me as I was not 'walking in her shoes'. I told her that I would still be the same person, I would just have the outer shell of a man. She said that she found that hard to accept because she believed that I would change and, not only that, she didn't like men's bodies.

After talking more, she said that she really wanted to stay in the relationship because she loved me, but that it was going to be very hard for her. We decided that we would just take things step by step and that we would continue to talk to each other about our feelings.

I was happy with how I felt and looked whist wearing the prosthetic, but then began to consider the reality of using men's toilets. Not only would I need to navigate using the opposing toilets to those of my birth gender, I would also have to factor in using a urinal with my new extension. I had practiced at home, but it was going to be very a very different experience at a urinal. I was excited to try it out, but also extremely nervous.

Would the men in the toilets be looking at me? Would they notice that my willy wasn't attached and that it looked unnatural? One thing I should mention at this point is that when I purchased this willy, I chose a colour that I thought most suited my skin tone. However, when it arrived, the colour was clearly not right for me. I knew that men's natal (born as male) willies were a darker colour to the rest of their skin, but there was quite a noticeable difference in the colour of this to the colour of my skin. I kept telling myself that they would not be looking at another man's 'bits', they would be getting on with their own business. I suppose these thoughts were there because of my insecurity, as I knew that the willy didn't look like part of me; I thought they might question me or, worse still, cause a scene. I also had to consider the fact that I was still a woman. Yes, I had short hair and wore men's clothing, but I was still a woman. Would people stare at me or, even worse, question me about why I was going into the men's toilets? Would they redirect me to the ladies' toilets? What if the cubicle was out of order and I was forced to use the urinal, even though I wasn't ready for that?

I would like you, for one moment, to try to put yourself in that position; how would you feel about using different toilets to those you had used all your life? How would you feel if you had to try to pee through a silicone tube that wasn't attached to your body, whilst making it look as if you had been doing this all your life? How would you feel if people questioned you on your choice of toilets? Can you imagine the anxiety that this might cause?

A little later on in my transition, one of the things I learned about when talking to friends, was that there are actually unspoken rules used in men's toilets. Firstly, men don't tend to talk to each other unless they are friends and even then, generally, they don't. On the other hand, women will happily chat away in next-door cubicles. Secondly, when men walk into the toilet, they pay close attention to the layout of the urinals and, apparently, this is so they can work out which urinal is best for them to use. Let's say there are three urinals and the two outer urinals are already occupied, leaving the remaining vacant urinal (in the middle) free. It seems that the general behaviour is a reluctance to use that vacant one in between. It is almost as though there is an invisible boundary that needs to be observed. Also, more importantly, men do not stand there and stare at other men's 'bits'. I wish I had known all of this at the start because I wouldn't have felt so scared.

As I previously mentioned, I had also purchased a chest binder from the same company as the prosthetic willy. A binder is a tight vest/top that is specifically designed for females that wish to have a masculine looking chest. It incorporates panels that are made of a material that flattens the breasts. The binders are made to be extremely tight, which makes them uncomfortable to wear for long periods of time, especially for people with larger chests.

There are guidelines on how long someone should wear a binder as they can cause injuries to the chest, such as permanent deformation of the breasts or constriction of the lungs. Another issue with binders is that wearing one during the summer months can be very unpleasant. They generally have an extra layer of material which can make the wearer hot and sweaty.

Given the fact that binders can be dangerous if worn for too long, many people have to take them off for periods of time which can cause 'body dysphoria' or 'body dysmorphia', a condition that makes a person worry about certain parts of their body and feel shame and embarrassment. Some people choose to ignore the advice on how long a binder should be worn, because they cannot bear to see themselves without one, or for anyone else to see them without one. Fortunately, proper binders are now available as, when they weren't, people would bind their chests with constrictive bandages which could be even more dangerous than the more modern binders.

Chapter Three - One Size Fits All?

I began to research more about being Transgender (Trans), what it meant and what it actually looked like. I very quickly realised that there is so much diversity amongst the Trans community - there is no such thing as 'one size fits all'.

I looked at other people's stories on YouTube and purchased a book entitled 'Transgender 101'. This book was of great value to me as it explained, in simple terms, what it means to be Transgender. It wasn't a story of anyone's life, but was more a factual analysis. I learned that there were several things to consider about my future, about how I wanted to look and how that would make me feel. There were so many decisions that I would need to make, for example, when and who should I tell ('coming out'), changing my name legally, choosing a new name, starting hormone therapy, what surgeries, if any, did I want and so many more.

What struck me most at that time was, which other 'normal' adult has to make these life-altering decisions? Why did I have to make these decisions to be able to live my life happily? I felt angry, scared, confused and alone.

After a period of time, probably no more than a week, I began to feel a little more positive. I had been doing some more research and I was quickly realising that I was most definitely not on my own, and that there would be support for me, if and when I needed it.

I was now 75% to 80% certain that I wanted to begin the process of transitioning fully from female to male. I knew with some clarity that, for me to truly be me, I would need to transition medically, with the aid of hormone therapy. Testosterone therapy would bring changes in my hormone levels so that Oestrogen was no longer the dominant hormone. I learned about the changes that hormone therapy, in the short-term, would bring, and this included a deepening of the voice and the growth of facial and other body hair. In the longer-term, this therapy would bring changes to fat distribution in certain areas of my body, creating a more masculine looking jaw-line and slimmer hips. Unfortunately, I would take on a more masculine-looking belly, commonly known as a 'beer-belly'. This was not something that I looked forward to, but it would be part of the expected changes.

I also learned that I would need to have multiple surgeries to physically change my body in all the places that were female. I was excited at the prospect of becoming me, but I also worried about the consequences of the long-term irreversible effects that surgery would have on my body. What would happen if I changed my mind; would it be too late? Would I then have to live the rest of my life stuck in a body I didn't want to be in? At this point, I asked myself the question, would this be any worse than continuing to live in the body I was born in, and the answer to that, was a resounding NO!

I looked online for sites where I could find information about the surgeries I may face further down the line.

I noticed that there was a lot more information available about male to female transition than there was the other way around. I did, however, find some sites giving information and some detailed and very graphic images of surgery. This was informative, but so scary! To think that I would have to go through all that, just to become someone that I should have been all my life. It just didn't seem fair to me; why wasn't I born a boy? I did have doubts, and who in their right mind wouldn't, but I had to ask myself if I could I ever be happy without it. Could I live my life in my chosen role without this surgery and just medically transition with Testosterone? I was confused and slightly disturbed at the prospect of full transition.

I knew that I was going to need some support, as I felt scared and alone with these scary thoughts. I felt that I needed to be around like-minded people who were going through the same thing as me or that had already been through it. I searched the Internet and found a support Group called TG-Pals. I looked at their website and, immediately, I realised I had found a really friendly, laid-back and supportive group. I learned that they held group gatherings twice a month and that seemed perfect for me.

It took me a little while to pluck up the courage to go to a meeting as I am quite a shy person. The thought of going to meet a lot of new people, not knowing what to expect, was definitely out of my comfort zone. However, I managed to get to my first meeting and I was so pleased that I did. What an eye-opener it was to meet so many lovely people. They were all in different stages of transition, some were not transitioning at all for various reasons, but were there because they still wanted to dress and look the way they needed to and wanted to. The group was set up as a safe space for people to explore their identities in whichever way they chose.

During my first meeting, I was introduced to a post-operative 'trans' man. His situation was slightly different to mine, as when he met his partner, he had already begun the transition process and his partner knew him as a man from the very beginning. When I talked to him, he confirmed that this had made his journey easier.

He was a great guy and he answered every single question that I threw at him. I even asked for a sneaky peak at his top and bottom surgeries! This was purely to satisfy my curiosity, and to educate myself a little more in the process and what to expect. He was so accommodating and trusting of me and I will always be grateful to him for that.

When I saw what he had, I was stunned and amazed by the work of the surgeons. But what struck me most was what he had been through to get to this point; I was in awe of him. I remember saying to him that he was a brave man to have gone through all of those complicated and painful surgeries. He told me that he didn't feel brave, it was just something that he had to do. Now that I have transitioned, I can relate to what he said. People often tell me how brave I am and I always say the same thing, I am not brave, I just had to do it. I can see why others may think it brave but, to the individual, there is no choice.

After meeting him, I was 85%-90% sure that this was the right decision for me. I want to thank him from the bottom of my heart, as he was truly amazing with me and I will never forget the care he showed me at such a pivotal point in my transition.

I also met a young lad at TG-Pals who was born a girl, but knew from a very young age, that he was in the wrong body. He had come along to the meeting with his Mum and he had the full support of his family. I really liked him and we got on well, so much so, that we became friends. Over a period of time, I seemed to take on a sort of mentor role and he felt comfortable talking to me about himself. Sometime later, I met the rest of his family, his Dad and younger Brother and we all became friends.

I became so proud of him as he knew exactly how he felt, what he wanted and how he was going to achieve it; he was definitely more grown-up than his years. His family were amazing and gave him 100% support.

Let's rewind things a little so that I can explain in more detail about the processes involved in the early stages of my transition….

In July 2012, my GP referred me to the local mental health team, so that they could make an assessment of my mental state. They took a detailed history, and then asked about my aspirations.

I was told that they needed to decide whether I was of sound mind and capable of making a decision about transitioning. This is a very crucial and necessary step in the process as, when the assessment was finished, they concluded that I was of sound mind (little did they know of the underlying 'streak of insanity' that runs through our family)!

A few months passed and I hadn't heard anything at all about my referral from the GP to the GIC. I made some enquiries and found out that they hadn't received a referral for me. Unfortunately, this delay put me two months behind. I contacted the GIC and they, eventually, told me that they had found the referral letter, which I can only assume meant that they had lost it in the first place. I asked if they could move me further along the waiting list, but they said that I would just have to wait my turn. I had read about the extremely long waiting lists for consultations and surgeries and I was annoyed that my letter had been lost, but there was nothing I could do about it, I just had to be patient.

I was now at the stage where I was beginning to research the process of changing my name by Deed Poll. I looked at the Deed Poll website and downloaded the relevant forms that I would need to complete. I had decided that it was the right time to take on my new identity and, having given it some thought, I chose my new name. In early September 2012, I signed the legal documents to enable the change of name. This documentation had to be signed by an independent witness in a certain profession, for example, a member of the Police or a solicitor.

I had to wait a while for this process to be completed, but when I received my official Deed Poll Certificate, I was so happy. It was not only the recognition of my new name, it was also recognition of me being male and that was such a proud moment for me. It was as if I had been given official confirmation that I could begin my new life. Now that I had the Deed Poll Certificate, I began sending out certified copies to all the relevant authorities and companies with which I had accounts. This process was extremely satisfying and it was the icing on the cake when I received confirmation addressed to Mr Daniel Canter.

I still hadn't heard from the GIC about the date of my first consultation and I was becoming impatient, so I decided to take matters into my own hands and researched the possibility of seeing a Gender Specialist privately. I knew that it would be expensive, but I couldn't wait any longer. It felt as though the door to my future fulfilment and happiness was locked and that someone else held the key. I needed get this process moving for my own sanity.

I needed to make sure that by going down the private treatment route, I would still be eligible for NHS funding when it came to the continuation of my medical and surgical transition. I found out that I would be able to remain on the NHS pathway for treatment, whilst also pursuing the private treatment route, and this would be achieved through what is called shared care. Once I was at the front of the NHS list, they would then take over my care and apply for the necessary funding for medical and surgical treatment. This would be dependent on the individual GP surgery, as the costs would come out of their budget.

I began to ask for recommendations for private treatment and was told about Gendercare. I made some initial enquiries and, after a about a week, a consultant made contact with me and offered me an appointment. Unfortunately, the private route can be rather expensive and therefore, not accessible to everyone. I didn't have loads of money, but I just had to get things started.

In Sept 2012, I had my first consultation at the Gendercare offices in London. I attended the appointment with my partner as she wanted to be there, not only for moral support, but also to enable her to understand what was to come for both of us.

The day of the appointment came and we made our way into London. On our arrival at the reception area, we were met by a kind-faced man who made me feel completely at ease. He took us through to his consulting room and told us a little about himself and what he does at the clinic. He took his own, very detailed history and listened very intently to what I had to say. He asked me if I had done anything up until that point to start the process of transitioning, for example, changing my name or telling anyone about it. He said that this was an important part of the social transition process and, without a period of social transition, I would not be considered for medical and surgical intervention. He explained that anyone wishing to transition has to live life as their chosen gender for at least two years before moving onto the next stages.

During the consultation I could see that my partner was struggling whilst she was listening to what I was saying. She was, however, able to be very open with the consultant about anything I may have forgotten to say. She also told him of the effect that this was having, and might continue to have, on our future relationship. I was extremely grateful that she was there with me as she was amazingly supportive.

After over an hour of history taking, the consultant told me that the floor was mine to ask any questions, no matter what they were. I had already written a list of all the things that I wanted to know and I began to go through it. He patiently answered all my questions, and he was able to put some of my fears aside; he told me that, in his opinion, I was definitely on the correct path. He also made it very clear that the journey ahead was not going to be an easy one and that it would involve both physical and emotional pain. He asked me if I had a good support system in place, because I was going to need it. Suddenly, this was all becoming very real.

At the end of the consultation, I was surprised to be given a diagnosis of Gender Dysphoria. I thought I would have to wait for the report to be sent to my GP, and then see my GP to get the diagnosis. I was so pleased to have received this so swiftly-it was the affirmation of my feelings that I so desperately needed.

The consultant told me that, following the consultation, he would send a report to my GP, and he also said that he would be sending the notes of the consultation to a private endocrinologist that works with him at Gendercare. He explained a little about the role of the endocrinologist in the process of transitioning, and that he would be responsible for determining whether I was a suitable candidate for hormone replacement therapy (Testosterone). He would also determine the type and the dosage.

I was now100% sure that I wanted to transition completely from female to male and made an appointment to see the endocrinologist at a hospital in Enfield. I was so excited, as this would be the appointment when I would be assessed for beginning the Testosterone hormone treatment, or 'T' as it is commonly called. This consultant asked his own series of questions and took his own detailed history, as this also served as a second opinion and confirmation of the original diagnosis.

At the end of the consultation, he said that he would definitely put me on T. He knew I was a smoker and he told me that I must give up smoking before I began taking it. He told me that men are at a higher risk of heart problems and other health-related issues if they smoke whilst using hormone therapy. I had already stopped smoking weeks before as I had already been told this by the first Gendercare physician. I assured him that I had stopped and he agreed to start me on T.

He explained about the different types of T that I could take and those most commonly used, and said that he thought that the best one for me would be in gel form.

I will explain in a little more detail about the different forms of T.

There are different brands of T and different routes by which they can be administered. The gel is topical (administered onto the skin). It is applied daily and for the rest of the person's life.

The other way that T can be given is via the IM (intramuscular injection) route. This can either be given by a nurse or the person can be taught to self-inject. The frequency and dosage are determined by the person's base levels of Oestradiol (Oestrogen) and Testosterone, which are calculated using the results of a blood test. Someone using IM injections would also have to be on them for life.

Both of these options require the Trans person to have regular blood tests. These tests are to monitor, not only the levels of Testosterone and Oestrogen in the body, but are also to ensure that vital organs, such as the liver and kidneys, are functioning well; these tests also check that the Testosterone is not having any adverse effect on them. Having spoken to others taking T, and through my own experience, I can tell you that there are pros and cons to consider when choosing the route of application, and I will talk about these below:

The pros for using gel are:

* A simple application once daily, with no requirement to visit a nurse

*When Testosterone enters the body via the skin, it is absorbed differently and gives a continuous dose, so there are no peaks and troughs (dips) in levels.

*The changes to the body are gradual, giving time to adjust. This is particularly noticeable as there is a direct effect on the vocal cords, demonstrated by a deepening of the voice. Because it is not a sudden change, it allows for a more well-rounded vocal range. The vocal range in men is lower than in women and this is due to the thickness of the vocal folds. When people begin taking T, the vocal folds become thicker, deepening the voice. If this happens too quickly, it doesn't allow as much time for the vocal folds to thicken and the person can end up with a more limited vocal range.

The cons for using gel are:

*Some people find that daily application can be tedious and could be forgotten.

*Some of the gel can be transferred from the person to a partner and/or any pets in the household. I'm sure you might imagine the effects of passing on male hormones to a woman but, one could assume with some certainty, that facial hair would be one of the undesired effects. Also, transferring a human hormone medication to pets would be unsafe.

*Some people also say that they didn't feel as though the changes happened quickly enough for them and they ended up switching from gel to injections.

The pros for IM injections:

*The changes can happen relatively quickly which, for some, is what they need. The dosage levels are monitored via blood tests and are adjusted according to the results.

*The injections are given weeks apart and this means that the person doesn't have to apply gel daily. The frequency of these injections is dependent on blood test results and the brand of T being given.

The cons for IM injections:

*The IM injections can be very painful. Because the injections are given straight into a muscle, they have to be administered slowly. The pain can last for a few hours and can also cause the legs to go numb.

*The levels go through a peak and trough cycle, so this means that when the injection is first given, the person's Testosterone level will spike. As the effects begin to wear off, the level of Testosterone will dip, which can cause lethargy, moodiness, anxiety and depression. Not everyone will experience these symptoms, but they are quite common.

Chapter Four - Pot of Gold

I was beginning to accept the realities of my journey, and I started to tell more and more people about who I was- the real me. I told extended family, neighbours, friends, and my boss at work. They all reacted so positively, which made me feel loved and cared for. They told me that no matter what I did to change my body, they would still love me and be there to support me.

I spoke to my boss; she was great and told me not to worry about anything at work. She told me that they would support me in any way they could. She also told me, in no uncertain terms, that bullying in any form, whether it be by customers or my colleagues, would not be tolerated. She asked me which toilets I would prefer to use and I said that I would use the disabled one as I was not yet comfortable enough to use the men's toilets with colleagues that had known me before transition. She said that she couldn't imagine being in my position and that she would do everything she could to make me comfortable when I was at work.

We had a very light-hearted discussion about my transition, which made me feel comfortable and at ease, and I felt that I would have her full support. She asked me how I would like to proceed and asked if I would like her to start the process of telling the other managers within the store.

I said that I was happy for her to tell the managers, and that I would begin telling my colleagues.

Looking back, I don't think I realised the scale of what was to come, as there were over three hundred staff that worked in that store and I would be changing from a woman to a man in front of their eyes. Because I felt I would be supported, I thought I would be ok and I was able to take it in my stride. As time went on, I began to feel more confident and I felt able to smile at the prospect of living the rest of my life happily in the gender in which I should have been born.

Following my disclosure at work, I had an overwhelming amount of support, understanding and questions; there were so many questions!! But I felt pleased that people were asking those questions because it meant that they were genuinely interested; either that or they were very curious. In either way, it gave me the opportunity to talk to them about my feelings and how things would begin to change for me. If, like me, they had never heard the word Transgender, nor met anyone that was Transgender, it was a way of me helping them to understand the emotions and feelings that someone might experience. Also, I could explain the processes involved in transitioning so that, should they ever encounter someone else who felt the same, they might have empathy and understanding toward that person.

Life at work was good and I continued to tell many people. For the most part, there was nothing but acceptance. There was only ever one situation, to my knowledge, that was negative. It was whilst on a break in the canteen when

I overheard a colleague talking about someone in their family that was male, but wanted to be female. I couldn't hear everything that was being said, but from what I could hear, my colleague and his family were extremely against it. They didn't understand why and they were extremely embarrassed by this person. I did hear some laughter coming from the people on that table and I made the assumption that this was because he was making fun of this family member.

At the time, I shrugged it off and carried on with my break. It wasn't until I walked out of the canteen and one of the section managers asked me to go into one of the meeting rooms, that I began to realise that the conversation had actually had an impact on me.

The manager asked me if I was okay and said that he had overheard the conversation. I told him that I hadn't heard everything, but what I had heard upset me a little. I also told him that now I was scared at the prospect that once he found out about me, he would be talking about me behind my back or, even worse, that he may bully me. My manager said that he would be speaking to this person and that I should try not to worry, as they would not tolerate any kind of harassment or bullying. I was extremely grateful to him and felt that he genuinely cared about me.

About a week later, the aforementioned colleague approached me on the shop floor and apologised to me. He told me that it was his father-in-law that he was talking about that day in the canteen. He then went on to tell me the back-story and the family's feelings around him wanting to transition to female. I listened to him before I said anything because I wanted to hear the full story. It was actually about a lack of understanding of what that person was going through. I didn't want to give any advice, I just wanted him to hear my story so that he might have a better understanding.

When we finished talking, he thanked me for being so open with him and said that he now better understood what his father-in-law might be feeling. He said he also now felt more comfortable when talking to him and was trying to offer some support. I felt good about this because, what had begun as an unpleasant situation turned into a positive one and gave us both a new and better understanding of each other.

As time went on, my partner and I began to have even more concerns about how my transition would affect our relationship. I battled with the fact that I didn't want her to go on the journey with me because there would be so much uncertainty, post-transition. Transition posed so many unanswered questions for both of us and neither of us knew how things would be.

So many things were going on that I felt insecure and a failure, not only to me but also to her. I still couldn't seem to communicate with her, even though she had been nothing but supportive of me. I became selfish and consumed by everything that was going on for me, but I failed to see what she was going through. However, we still tried to continue with some semblance of a 'normal' relationship.

The time came for me to go to the pharmacy to collect my first prescription; I was so excited, but I was also a little nervous. Would I be questioned, looked at strangely? Here was I, a woman, going into a pharmacy to collect a male hormone. When the pharmacist handed it to me, there were no strange looks or questions, he just explained the dosage and I went on my merry way. What I had in my hands represented a pot of gold, and I held on to it as if it were just that. This little box, containing 31 perfect little tubes of Testim® (one of the gel brands) was the first key, in a figurative bunch, that was going to unlock my future! I started to use the T every day and was amazed at how this made me feel. I knew that the effects wouldn't kick-in for some time, but just applying it made me feel powerful and in control of my destiny.

I had been struggling with my image and with people's perception of my gender. I was sometimes called Sir, but people would often correct themselves once they realised, usually after they had heard me speak, and this embarrassed me. I would sometimes hear children say to their mother or father, "that man over there" but then they would be wrongly corrected and told, "no, that's a woman"

I noticed that children seemed to have so much more foresight or intuition. They seemed to be able to perceive what was right in front of them. Maybe this is because they were still young and were yet to be moulded by society into what were the stereotypical 'norms', and this made me angry and embarrassed. I would have to hold myself back from saying, 'listen to your child, they are right and you are wrong', however I didn't ever say it as I didn't want to draw extra attention to myself. In hindsight, what was I expecting? Rightly or wrongly, they were gendering me on what they could see or hear.

Unfortunately, my relationship was really beginning to go downhill rapidly, and we both decided that it would be better if we went our separate ways. I had reached a point where I was hurtling at a hundred miles an hour into my new future and I was completely closed down as to how she was feeling. I was so scared that I would lose her from my life completely after everything we had been through together.

Because we still loved each other and neither of us wanted to lose the other, we agreed that we would give each other some space and that maybe, in time, we could continue our friendship; I wanted that more than anything. This woman had thrown me a life-line and, without her, I am not sure I would have been in this position now, writing this book. Please don't misunderstand, at no point was I ever suicidal, but I was spiralling down into a pretty dark hole and she was the one that reached down into that hole and pulled me out.

I still hadn't heard anything from the GIC regarding my appointment and I knew that I couldn't afford to self-fund indefinitely. Fortunately, I was able to get another prescription without having to have another consultation, but this was on the proviso that I would have some blood tests done. I was so grateful for that, as each consultation cost approximately £250. I had the blood tests done and awaited the results. I remember thinking could this gel that I rub on my skin once a day, really change my hormone levels so dramatically? The answer was, yes it could and it had. The results showed that my T levels were 20 (a good therapeutic level), and my Oestradiol levels had dropped significantly; I was thrilled!

As time went on, I began to realise that continuing to self-fund would not be possible. I had now moved into my own flat and had become completely self-sufficient, so money was tighter than ever. I contacted my GP to ask if she would take over the responsibility for my blood-tests and prescribing T. After a telephone discussion, she said that she would need a care plan from my consultant and then she would need to look at the GP practice's funding in order to commit to this. I told her that I would contact Gendercare and ask them to provide her with my care-plan and then she could take it from there.

I was beginning to feel more confident about my image. I had started to cultivate small patches of stubble on my chin and, although this growth was extremely patchy, it gave me such a confidence boost. Ironically though, I was called madam even more than I was pre-T. This hurt my feelings because it felt as though people just couldn't see me. I thought that I conformed to most of the prerequisites of being male. I had the swagger, the clothes, the stubble and, possibly, the attitude. Why couldn't they see me?

I was enjoying and valuing the peer support that I had found in TG-Pals; these people enriched my life in so many ways. One of the great things that TG-Pals offers is one-to-one support through mentoring. This was good for me as I am better in one-to-one scenarios than I am with larger groups. I also went out to a popular gay venue as myself, Daniel, and this was the first time I had done this. This was a liberating experience and showed me that I could socialise without fear of being judged. I did still have a lot of unanswered questions which led to some confusion, but I decided to just let it be. I would find the answers to these questions when the time was right. I didn't want to place restrictions and boundaries on myself because that wouldn't be productive - this journey was going to be one of exploration, not rules.

It is a well-known saying that 'Life begins at forty.' Well, I was nearly forty and felt like my 'real' life was just beginning.

Chapter Five - Confidence

At this point, there hadn't been many huge physical changes, other than the development of more facial and body hair. However, the psychological changes were profound. I was becoming much more confident in my appearance and was being mis-gendered much less. I was also no longer getting so many strange looks whilst out and about.

This was having a very positive effect on my emotional well-being. When people did slip up and mis-gender me, I found that, because I was more confident, it was becoming increasingly more difficult to be tolerant of those situations and I would have to bite my tongue more and more to suppress what I really wanted to say to them. Wasn't the facial hair enough for people to get it right? I had much more tolerance with friends and family, because they knew my former identity and former name (Nikki), so it was probably going to be a more difficult process for them. However, I was surprised, as they very rarely got it wrong.

People told me that my jaw-line had become more masculine. I couldn't say I had noticed that but I suppose because I saw myself every day, it was more difficult for me to see any subtle differences. I kept checking back on old photos to see if I could see any changes, and I couldn't see many. I had been working out to try to gain some muscle mass on my upper body to give me a more masculine physique. I was managing to achieve this but it was a slow process. I was lucky though, as I had a fairly masculine upper body already, with broad shoulders, so at least I had the right frame to begin with.

Rather unfortunately, the areas that hadn't changed were my hips, thighs and buttocks. I knew that, with the use of T, there would be some fat redistribution and that these areas would slowly begin to change, but I wanted this to happen quickly as these areas of my body had always caused some dysphoria.

I had begun to think about dating but I struggled to know into which bracket I would fit. Who would want to be with me? Would 'normal', straight women want to be with a Trans man? I was neither male nor female, so how could I identify myself, let alone ask someone else to attempt it? I decided that the best thing to do would be to just put myself out there, thinking what's the worst that can happen? Suddenly, I came to a very horrible realisation - there was a very strong possibility that I could be alone for the rest of my life. I wondered if I was alone in feeling this, but after talking to other Trans people, I have found out that it is actually very common to have these thoughts.

After some soul-searching, I decided that I would I introduce myself to the world of Trans-dating websites. I felt that this would be the best place to start, as I would be able to meet like-minded and like-bodied people who truly understood what it was to be transgender. The idea of dating another Trans person, was a strange one to me because I didn't really understand how I would fit in sexuality-wise, and it was confusing. Hopefully, at the very least, I would make some more Trans friends and then, if anything further developed, that would be a bonus.

I had now received the go-ahead from my GP and I was incorporated into the NHS Care Pathway. This meant that my GP surgery (overseen by the GIC) would take over my blood tests and the prescribing of T. I would be put on the waiting lists for all future surgical appointments.

I was so grateful that I was being supported by the NHS in my journey to become my true self because anyone going through transition in another country would have to fund the process themselves. However, unpredictable waiting times, cancelled appointments and an overstretched and under-funded service would be some of the issues that I might have to deal with. When I looked at the figures produced by the clinic about how many patients were on their lists, I knew that it was going to be a long and bumpy road.

I had come across resistance from some people about whether the NHS should fund the transition process. This way of thinking was only aired by a small minority, but those people didn't think that the NHS should 'foot the bill'. They said that it was each person's choice to transition. Whenever I encountered this, I became angry and asked them why should people seeking help with alcoholism, drug addiction, smoking cessation and weight management be entitled to NHS-funded treatment, but not someone that needed to change their body due to gender dysphoria? Being Transgender is not a choice, some people are born that way and those that are, suffer horrendously, both emotionally and physically! I am not saying that people should not be entitled to treatment for the aforementioned issues, but no-one should stand in judgement over who should have that entitlement. Everyone should have the right to access the NHS whenever their physical or emotional health is at risk.

I attended Trans Pride in Brighton that year with my ex-partner. It was a first for me and only the second year that it had been running. We were shown around by a lady who lived in Brighton who I had met on one of the Trans Internet groups. She had been to the event in the previous year and she agreed to be our guide. It was a relatively small affair with a main stage, a bar and some stalls representing local Trans groups. The event was tiny in comparison with Gay Pride, but I had a feeling it would grow year-on-year. Brighton was definitely the right place to host it as the town has a really chilled-out vibe; the diversity there has always been noticeable and, for that reason, it attracts varied types of people. There was a huge sense of camaraderie, as we were all there because we all identified differently from our birth gender. I want to explain that not everyone who identifies as Transgender will transition. Transgender is an umbrella word used to describe all different ways of identifying.

Below is a representation of the Transgender Umbrella
(Image created by Tyler Kennett)

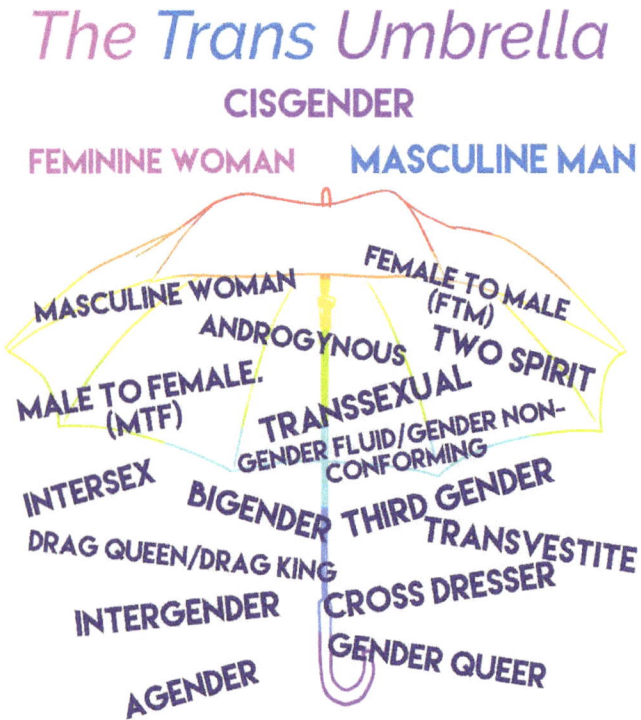

The Trans Umbrella

CISGENDER

FEMININE WOMAN   MASCULINE MAN

MASCULINE WOMAN
FEMALE TO MALE (FTM)
ANDROGYNOUS
TWO SPIRIT
MALE TO FEMALE (MTF)
TRANSSEXUAL
GENDER FLUID/GENDER NON-CONFORMING
INTERSEX
BIGENDER
THIRD GENDER
DRAG QUEEN/DRAG KING
TRANSVESTITE
CROSS DRESSER
INTERGENDER
GENDER QUEER
AGENDER

Chapter Six - Born in the Wrong Box

I was eagerly awaiting my next appointment at the GIC, as it would be my first consultation for chest surgery. This was the first surgical step in altering my physical appearance and, in some ways, the most important. To be able to have a masculine chest and walk around with no top on was so important to me.

The consultation date in November 2013 finally arrived, and I was seen at the GIC by a consultant for the first appointment in the process of being signed off for chest surgery. The appointment went really well and the consultant decided that I should proceed to the next stage of referral for this procedure, as every surgery had to be signed off by two clinicians.

During my consultation I was asked if I was a smoker. I am not a good liar so, when asked if I had stopped smoking, my reaction was to tell the truth and admit that I had stopped but, also, to say that due to some stressful circumstances, I had begun again and smoked occasionally. I was told, in no uncertain terms, that I had to stop smoking and, if I didn't, they would not endorse continuation to surgery. The doctors are very clear about their clinical obligation to make their patients aware of the risks involved. I was told that I would be endorsed for surgery on the proviso that I stopped immediately. If I couldn't do this, then my next consultation wouldn't go ahead until I could. Needless to say, I stopped, pretty much straight away. I didn't want anything getting in the way of me progressing to surgery.

My next appointment was scheduled for June 2014, however, due to the clinician being unwell on that day, it was postponed until Sept 2014. This was a real blow, as I had been waiting so long for it to then be cancelled at the last minute. I would have to wait another three months!

Finally, the appointment date arrived! I was asked by the clinician, why I had been waiting for so long? I told her that my last appointment was rescheduled as she had been unwell. She apologised and said that, hopefully, things would be a little smoother from then on. At the end of the consultation, she advised me that she would be endorsing my chest surgery and that she would also be referring me for the next stage, which would be genital surgery. I was so excited when she said that she would be endorsing the chest surgery and, even more so when I realised she would also endorse my genital surgery.

I moved out of the place that I rented as I was struggling to pay all the bills on my own. My former partner and I had continued to build on our friendship and she, very kindly, invited me to move back in with her so that I could save some money. I was extremely grateful to her for this as I am not sure how I would have coped. After I had lived with her for a while, she and I and another friend, went on a fantastic holiday to Egypt. During the holiday, I started to think about living with her. I was so grateful that she had given me a safe place to stay, but I felt that it was not fair to her to have me around all the time. She needed to move on with her life and having me there was making things difficult. When we got back from our holiday, we talked and it was decided that I should move out so that we could both have the freedom and space we needed to move on with our lives.

I moved into a lovely place in a country village, just outside Sittingbourne, in Kent. It was a converted stable that was originally inhabited by a master huntsman. The stable was tiny, but it had everything I needed and the rent and bills were affordable. This little haven became affectionately known as 'The Hut'. The main house, to which the hut was attached, was named 'the cottage' after being referenced by Jane Austen in one of her books, 'Persuasion', and it dated back to the 17th Century. It was a stunning building that was surrounded by a few acres of land and was bordered by open expanses of fields and forest. I had my own private garden which was beautiful and full of unique and charming characteristics. That little garden became my favourite place to be and I spent many hours gardening there and making it my own little piece of heaven

The landlady, who was in her late 70s, looked after the majority of the house and land herself and this included looking after 2 ponies, a donkey and her three cats. The ponies and donkey were not hers; they were owned by a neighbour. They had an arrangement between them, that she would house them in her stables and on her land and look after them and, in return, her neighbour would do her ironing for her- I thought this was such a fantastic arrangement!

My landlady was an amazing and lovely lady, and we very quickly built up a friendship. I had to go to the main house to shower and do my washing-up as The Hut didn't have running water, and we would often chat and drink Bailey's coffee together in her country kitchen, in the company of her three Persian cats. You may remember that I mentioned, earlier in my story, about a lady that said to me that I had been 'born in the wrong box' after I had told her that I wanted to transition- she was that lady.

I had decided to tell her about my transition because I knew that, at some point, I would be having surgery and that I would have to leave her house and move back in with my parents during my recovery. When I told her my thoughts, I remember feeling quite overwhelmed at her response- she simply said "You cannot help the fact that you were born in the wrong box". I thought that was such a brilliant way to look at it. She was so forward-thinking and non-judgemental and she, just simply, accepted me for who I was.

When I received the referral for my chest surgery, I was asked to call the secretary to arrange the date for this. I had already chosen my consultant based on some pictures I had seen online, showing his results and I had also read some referrals made by other Trans guys. This particular consultant was based at a hospital in Brighton. I spoke to his secretary and everything was very straightforward and, by the end of the conversation, we had set a date-April 15th 2015.

I was absolutely thrilled that this was happening - finally I would have a masculine chest. I would be able to fulfil that compelling deep-routed need to walk around without wearing a top, situation dependant, of course.

As I've already mentioned, I had been looking at some Trans dating sites, in the hope that I might eventually meet someone. I had started to talk to a woman on one particular site and over a period of time we had been getting to know one another. We just seemed to click and we were able to talk so freely and easily about our feelings of being born in the wrong body. We had so much in common and we both found we had a real appreciation and understanding of each other's past and present lives. Had I found someone who could be a potential partner – perhaps someone who had an understanding of what I was going through? I was so happy!

We continued to chat, online, for a while before agreeing to meet. I wanted to make sure that we were 'on the same page' and, to say that I was nervous would be an understatement! We agreed to meet at a pub and decided that we would wait for each other in the car park.

I already knew that I was attracted to her because I had seen her profile photos, but when I saw her in the car park, she was even more beautiful! I became even more nervous, as I wasn't sure if I would live up to her expectations. We walked into the pub, I bought her a drink and we sat down at a little secluded table; I was beginning to feel more at ease. The conversation just seemed to flow so well and everything felt natural and comfortable. We sat for a few hours and we talked more about our lives and the commonalities of our journeys. We both said that it felt as if we had each met someone that truly understood us. At the end of the afternoon, we arranged to see each other again, and then we went on our separate ways.

We had already worked out that the distance between us and our differing shift patterns would mean that we would have to be creative when it came to planning time together. But we would make it work somehow. Over a period of time, we became very close in all aspects of a 'normal' healthy relationship. But the one thing that was missing was a deeper intimacy. We had always talked openly and honestly about our bodies, how we felt about them and how they affected each of us psychologically; I knew that when it came to the point of physical intimacy, it would be a struggle for her. I also knew that we were in different places when it came to the psychological impact that our body dysphoria had on each of us.

Certain areas of my body affected me greatly, but I had come to terms with the fact that, until it changed, I wouldn't let it hold me back during intimate experiences. Unfortunately, her issues around sexual intimacy were more deeply rooted and this caused her a lot of anxiety. Even though I knew her feelings about intimacy, I thought that we had every chance of building a successful and happy relationship.

My next medical appointment, which was to discuss genital surgery, was scheduled for April 2015. But in an unusual and happy twist of fate, that appointment was cancelled and brought forward, and so I was seen in February 2015 instead. At this appointment, I was hoping to get my first genital surgery signature. When I arrived at the consultant's office, the first thing he said to me was, "So you are here for your second genital surgery signature". Well, that threw me, as I'd thought I would have to have another appointment to get to that stage. I then recalled being told at my last appointment, that the next steps would, hopefully, be a lot smoother. The last consultant had actually given me my first signature for genital surgery- I was a very happy bunny!

At this appointment, we discussed why I wanted and needed to have genital surgery. We also discussed briefly, the available procedures. He told me that there were two main procedures, one being Metoidioplasty, also known as 'Meta' and the second being Phalloplasty, also known as 'Phallo'

Meta, is a procedure that uses the clitoris (which will have grown when taking T) to create a functional and sensate penis. Aesthetically and functionally, it falls short, literally, as it is quite small. It is not really ever going to be big enough for penetrative sex and, also, not long enough to clear the fly when trying to pee standing up. Even though the clitoris grows somewhat when taking Testosterone, it will only grow to around 2-3" when erect. The benefits of having this procedure would be that you would retain all the sexual sensations that you had previously. This is because the surgeons don't interfere too much with it, other than to release it at the bottom so that it hangs a little more like a biological penis.

Phallo, is a procedure whereby surgeons make a penis that looks cosmetically appealing, is sensate and is also functional. This is achieved by using skin and fat from another site on the body to create the penis which would then be attached to the pubic area. The desired outcomes are that the person would have sensation in the penis, they would be able to stand and urinate through it, and they would be able to use the penis for penetrative sex.

The consultant told me that if I was considering Phalloplasty and using the radial (lower) forearm as the donor site, I may need some electrolysis on my forearm. He explained that because the surgeon would take the skin from that area to make the body of the penis, and that the inside part of my arm would be used to make the urethra, I might need any hair on my arm removed.

I would need to see the surgeon before deciding which procedure to have, as he would need to assess a viable donor site. The choice of the donor site is not all down to the person, but if they would prefer to use the forearm, there must be adequate blood flow to that area. To check that blood flow, a Doppler test (an ultrasound scan that determines the movement and velocity, in this case, of blood) is sometimes used. The surgeon's preference would be to use the person's non-dominant arm, but it very much depends on the result of the Doppler test. Because the surgeon would be interfering with arteries and nerves, I was told that the risk would be that I could experience some or, worst case scenario, a total loss of function of that arm and or hand. This scared me but, even then, I thought that this was the procedure I was likely to choose.

At the end of the appointment, the consultant endorsed this surgery, and told me that I would be added to the surgical waiting list. He asked if I would like to be discharged from the GIC as they would no longer need to see me. I hesitated, as I thought that, without their support, I might feel out on a limb. He put my mind at ease and told me that I could be seen again there if needed it.

I was beginning to be able to visualise a happy and fulfilled life in a way that I have never been able to envisage before, and this continued to be my driving force. There are always risks in our normal everyday lives, and we are generally able to assess those risks and make decisions based upon the potential outcomes. Unfortunately, there are many unknown risks and decisions Trans people face when it comes to changing their bodies through gender-affirming medical and surgical interventions. Anyone who has made the decision to transition will know that the potential outcomes far outweigh the risks.

Chapter Seven –Swap Shop

I was beginning to experience a shift in my social life and I seemed to be losing friendships with some of the people that I considered to be my support network. I know that social circles change all the time but, on this journey, constant and ongoing support is crucial. I took friends' opinions relating to my transition very personally and I became defensive. How could they possibly begin to understand what I was going through? When I look back, I realise that they probably just didn't understand, and found it difficult to express their opinions or feelings; I realised that they were not being judgemental. I had pushed them away to protect myself.

Time moved a little further on, and my current relationship was beginning to struggle. The intimacy issues that I previously mentioned had begun to affect us. Because I was taking Testosterone, I had the sex drive of a teen-aged boy and it was difficult for me not being able to be intimate with her.

However, the bond we had ran far deeper than just a surface sexual relationship. I needed to feel wanted sexually, but she still struggled even though she knew how much it meant to me to feel wanted and needed in this way.

We talked at great length about our feelings and we both decided to take a step back from the sexual part of the relationship and just be friends. We would definitely be there for one another in a supportive way, and we were both happy with our decision.

I wanted to check on the progress of my surgical referral, so I called the Gender Identity Clinic. It was over a month since my consultation and, for my peace of mind, I thought it was worth a call. I eventually spoke to one of the receptionists who informed me that my referral had been processed but was pending funding approval. I was told that in order to speed things up, I could try writing to the referring clinician. I composed a letter in which I put forward my case and I hoped that this would expedite things a little. It was not a queue-jumping exercise, I just needed in place some financial plans and, also, to discuss my post-surgery recovery with my manager at work.

My ex-partner and I were still very close and continued to support each other as much as we could. We maintained a great friendship and possibly became even closer than we were when we were together. As time went on, I think we had both begun to realise what we could lose.

The time had come for me to have my pre-op assessments for the top surgery, which were to be carried out in the hospital in Brighton, where I would have the surgery. I travelled to Cobham to be nearer to the hospital and spent the night with my ex-partner. During that evening, we ended up having a long and frank discussion about our relationship and ended up agreeing to try again. We both wanted to give the relationship time to grow and blossom, rather than stop it in its tracks and never let it realise its potential. We couldn't predict the future when it came to our surgeries, but we knew that we wanted to be with each other.

On the day of my pre-op assessments, we travelled to Brighton early to avoid any potential delays. We arrived early enough to have a wander around the marina and have a quick drink in a local pub, for some Dutch courage, perhaps. After our drink, we made our way to the hospital and checked in at the reception area. I began to feel quite nervous, but I was comforted by knowing that my partner was by my side. We talked about what this appointment meant to me and I said that this was what I had been waiting for, it was finally real, it was happening.

This was the first time that I would meet the surgeon who would be carrying out my operation and, although I was nervous, I was also excited about meeting him.

One of the tests scheduled for that day, involved taking swabs from various areas of my body to check for MRSA (Methicillin-resistant Staphylococcus Aureus) also referred to as a 'super bug'. One of the swab-sites was my groin area and I wasn't particularly comfortable with a stranger seeing that part of my body, but I knew that I would have to get used to this as I would be having multiple surgeries in the future.

The hospital was lovely and had a very homely feel, not at all clinical. It reminded me more of a hotel than a hospital. Being in Brighton, it was surrounded by stunning countryside, and the windows in my room provided impressive views of the South Downs.

The staff members in each department we visited were so helpful and friendly, and they made me feel totally at ease. My nerves slipped away and the reality and excitement of the situation took their place.

I was called into the nurse's office so that she could take some medical history and then after that, blood tests and observations were done, including heart rate, temperature and blood pressure. Swabs were taken to check for MRSA. The nurse actually handed me the swab for my groin so that I could do it, and this made me feel better. Once the examination was complete, I was given a clean bill of health and I was told that there were no issues with proceeding to surgery, but this would be on the proviso that my blood tests were ok and that the swabs came back negative.

The next appointment on that day was only half an hour later and was with the surgeon. I remember feeling quite nervous again, but because he was friendly, down to earth and relaxed around me, my nervousness melted away. There was a female nurse present throughout the entire consultation for safeguarding.

The surgeon began by taking his own medical history from me and then he asked me to go behind the curtain so that he could look at my chest. I remember feeling extremely awkward and it must have shown on my face because he quickly reassured me and said that it wouldn't take long, he just needed to take a quick look to decide on the best procedure for me. The nurse came in with me and asked me to undress my top area and to sit on the edge of the bed. When the surgeon came in, he asked me to sit straight and to lift my arms up so that he could take a proper look; it was all over in under a minute and I was so relieved.

He told me that he would be using a procedure known as double-incision mastectomy. Having already researched this surgery, I knew a little bit about it. He explained that this particular surgery is for anyone who has a chest measurement larger than an A-cup. He explained that the procedure would involve making an incision beginning just under the armpit, from one side of my body to the other. He would remove my nipples, resize them by making the areolae smaller, and he would re-graft them in the place where they would normally be on a male chest. He advised me that I would be left with a very long scar under my nipples and that the sensation in my nipples would not be the same as before surgery because the nerves are damaged when they are removed.

For information purposes, there are other, less invasive, chest surgery procedures offered. These keyhole, or peri-areolar, procedures leave a far lower level of visible scarring and the patient is able to retain sensation in the nipples because they have not been completely removed. The less invasive route would always be a better option, both for recovery and retention of sensation. However, aesthetically, the double-incision procedure provides a much more male-shaped chest. This is because the surgeon can take the correct amount of tissue away and sculpt the chest in such a way as to create the natural contours of a male chest.

My partner and I were doing well and we both felt that we had developed an even closer bond since being back together. We even experienced our first, slightly deeper and more intimate physical encounter. Afterward, we talked at length about how it made us feel. She told me that she went through lots of emotions before, during and after it, but that she felt comfortable and not pressured by me throughout. She also told me that, previously, she would have had to dig deep to try to break through some of the protective walls she had built around her. She said that it now came much more naturally to her and that it was nowhere near as emotionally-charged as before; this allowed her to be totally present, and not just willing herself to get through it just to keep the other person happy.

Over the next few months, we spent as much time as we could together and continued to build on our relationship. During that time, we shared some more intimate experiences, but I couldn't help feeling that she was still uncomfortable. When we had talked previously, she had told me that she knew this would change after surgery, but she still felt very uncomfortable with her body, especially the lower parts. I certainly didn't want to pressure her into anything that made her feel uncomfortable, and I knew that it was a case of being patient.

We had always shared a similar sense of humour and had experienced some truly wonderful moments of clarity during which we knew we were so right for each other. It was commonplace for her to walk into the bathroom to find my prosthetic willy up-ended on the edge of the bathtub whilst I was in the bath. There would also be times when I would find her prosthetic boobs sitting perkily on a shelf; this was so normal to us and we laughed about it regularly. We often talked about how good it would be if the surgeons were able to take off her bits and attach them to me and vice-versa- like a swap shop. We could go into hospital together and after being put under anaesthetic they could swap our bits. We were very sure that this would be available at some point in the future.

Over the next few months, I noticed that we were hardly intimate at all. I could sense that she was still really uncomfortable with intimacy. I tried my best to understand this and support her through it, but it was difficult for me as I craved that intimacy. I didn't want to give up on us again, so I tried my best to put it out of my mind and concentrate on all the other fantastic things our relationship gave me.

Chapter Eight - Invasion of the Body Snatchers

On 15th April 2015 I was admitted to the Nuffield Hospital in Brighton the for my long-awaited chest surgery. I arrived a little early and I was excited, but nervous. Again, my partner was by my side and she made me feel at ease. I checked in at the reception desk and then sat in the waiting area.

The admission went so smoothly, and all the staff members were lovely and made me feel comfortable. I was shown to my room by one of the admission clerks and, once there, I was shown how to use the nurse call button.

I was then visited by a nurse who explained to me how I would be prepared for surgery, and I was told that I was the first on the surgeon's list. I was happy with that because it meant less waiting time to feel nervous and anxious.

Following that, my surgeon came in for a chat about the procedure and to do some artwork on my chest. I questioned why he had drawn two arrows, one above each breast. I asked if it was to remind him that he was operating on my chest and not any other part of my body. He laughed and said "actually, it is to make sure everyone knows where the surgery is happening" This filled me with confidence.

After this, the anaesthetist visited me, and asked if I had any questions or concerns regarding the anaesthetic. I told him that my only concern was feeling nauseous post-surgery, as I have a phobia about feeling sick or vomiting. He said that he would run an anti-emetic (anti-sickness) drug through the drip line in theatre, which made me feel happier.

Once I had been seen by everyone, I was asked to get into my hospital gown and TEDS- (Thrombo-Embolus Deterrent Stockings-to stop any potential blood clots).I was given the option of either wearing their lovely couture paper pants during surgery or to wear my own new or clean boxers- I opted for my own new boxers!

I didn't wait long before I was whisked away on my white chariot to the operating theatre. My partner was allowed to walk with me down to the operating room doors, but no further. I did ask whether she could come into theatre with me so that she could offer her artistic/aesthetic opinion but, oddly, they said no!

The team in the anaesthetic room was so friendly, and we were chatting about the pre-med they used. I told them that I used to be a veterinary nurse and that we used some of the same drugs on animals. The friendly chit-chat helped me to relax whist they placed an anaesthetic cannula in my hand. When they were ready to begin the process, they asked me to, slowly, count down from 10. I am not sure how far I got with that, but I think I only managed to about 7 and then it was 'lights out'.

When I awoke in the recovery room, I remember the nurses talking to me, but I had no idea what they were saying. I must have fallen asleep again, as the next time I woke,

I was back in my own room without any idea of how I had got there, and my partner was there waiting for me. We talked and joked for pretty much the entire afternoon. I wasn't in pain but I was uncomfortable, as the surgical team had placed a pressure bandage around my chest; this was to minimise any swelling and it had to be left in place for two weeks (apart from when the wound needed to be checked or the dressing changed). Movement was difficult because of bruising around the area, but for the most part I didn't experience much pain. My oxygen saturation level, blood pressure and heart rate were monitored at regular intervals and everything seemed to be fine.

I needed to pee and I decided that I would get up to do this whilst my partner was still there. I knew that I would need some help and I didn't want to risk it alone. I had been warned about feeling faint when I stood up which would be due to a possible drop in my blood pressure. My partner helped me to get out of bed and, very slowly, to my feet. I did begin to feel dizzy but managed to make it over to the visitors' chair so I could sit and rest. It was the most horrible feeling, as I felt as if I was going to pass out; I also felt extremely hot and nauseous. My partner called a nurse and I got a telling off for trying to get up without them. The nurse checked my blood pressure and by that time it was almost back to normal. With the help of the nurse, I eventually made it to the toilet.

I didn't sleep too well that night, which was strange because normally an anaesthetic would continue to have an effect long after 'coming round'! I was also on morphine, so the combination of the two should have been enough to knock an elephant off its feet. Every time I felt as though I was going to nod off to sleep, my body would twitch or jerk. When a nurse checked on me in the early hours of the morning, I was asked if I needed any pain relief. I had been told not to let the pain build up too much as it would be harder for them to control it, and they would have to give a larger dose of pain-killers. They use a scale of 0-10 to score it, 0 being no pain and 10 being the highest level of pain. I think, at that time, I scored it at around four, so she gave me some codeine and paracetamol to take together. Within about an hour, the pain was tolerable and, although I still couldn't sleep due to the twitching and jerking, I was able to rest. It wasn't until the next day when Mum visited, that she told me she has the same experience after anaesthesia. Perhaps I inherited it from her?

The surgeon and the anaesthetist visited me the next morning. The anaesthetist wanted to make sure I was doing well after the anaesthetic, and the surgeon wanted to take off some of the pressure bandages to check for swelling and any leakage of the wound. All seemed well and it felt so nice to have the pressure released a little, even if it was only for a while. He said that everything had gone very well and that he was very happy with the result; he hoped that I would be also. He asked me if I had been working out as I had a pretty good set of 'pecs'. I said that I had been working on my upper body for a while as I wanted to achieve the best results I could. He said that this had paid off and that he really didn't have to do too much in the way of sculpting to achieve a male looking chest- I was thrilled! After the surgeon left the room, a nurse came to wrap me in another pressure bandage; I hadn't yet seen my chest properly, although, I could see that it looked flatter.

I was due to be discharged that morning at about 10am and I was waiting for the physiotherapist to arrive to show me some post-operative, mobilisation exercises. Following this visit, the nurse that I had met at my pre-admission appointment came to give me my discharge pack, which included pain-relief medication and some extra dressing materials.

My partner drove me to my parents' house and, fortunately, I didn't suffer too much pain during the journey as I had been given some Oramorph (oral morphine) before leaving the hospital, just to make me feel more comfortable.

Once with my parents, I was able to relax and begin the process of gaining strength and mobility.

I was advised to wear a sports binder to make sure that the pressure was maintained over the wounds.

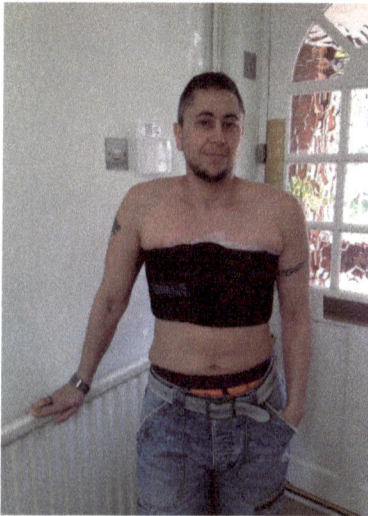

This is a picture of the chest binder I had to wear. It was actually a sports brace but worked really well.

I found it quite hard to get myself in and out bed at first and I needed a lot of assistance. However, it became easier after a few days. I slept in an almost upright position for the first week, not for any reason other than it was easier to get out of bed from that position rather than from a horizontal position.

A week later, I visited the hospital in Brighton for my post-op check; I also had the staples removed from my nipples. My appointment went very well overall, apart from feeling faint when both the surgeon and the nurse were pulling off the dressings.

I saw my chest properly for the first time and when I looked in the mirror, I was amazed- the results were far better than I had ever imagined they would be. I could see my 'pecs' and that made me smile. I was still feeling a little faint, but I wanted my partner to take some photos for me, also the surgeon wanted to take some pictures for his results portfolio.

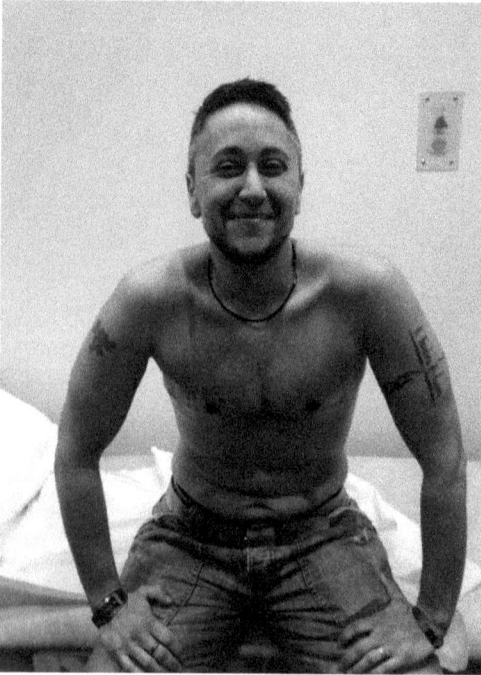

Chest Reveal- Happy boy

As you can see, the results are amazing and I was so happy-
I think the smile says it all!

I was told to wean myself off wearing the pressure binder
and to wear it mainly when I went out to give me some
support and protection. I was given a roll of medical
adhesive tape to put over the wounds excluding the nipples,
as they needed to have some ventilation to encourage
healing.

Having nothing on my chest was the most bizarre feeling as
I had worn a binder in some form or another for a few

years. I felt naked and I felt as though I should have been covering up, but It was a wonderful feeling to be able to sit with an open shirt and not be worried about my chest.

Some time passed and I was recovering well at my parents' house. I had a lot of time on my hands, and I began to think more and more about the relationship I was in. I was so much further along in my transition than she was, and I was concerned that I would not be able to maintain a non-sexual relationship with her. I knew that we needed to talk and we agreed to meet and to have coffee. We talked very openly, as we always had, about our feelings toward each other and, as it turned out, she was feeling the same way. We both felt that we would be better off as friends.

After I had recovered more, I left my parents' house and returned to The Hut in Kent. I didn't need any further help after the surgery, so it seemed like the right time to return.

I managed to return to work after about six weeks and I asked to be put on restricted duties. I had already spoken to my manager about this, so it was not a problem. I had to be very careful with my chest to ensure that I didn't do anything that would overstretch my capabilities. A bilateral mastectomy is quite an invasive procedure and, as with any invasive surgery, it is important to allow a sufficient period of time to heal. If the scars are stretched early on in the healing process, this can leave a thicker scar-line, and I didn't want that to happen.

Chapter Nine - Love

The next phase of 'operation change' was in progress. I was still awaiting authorisation of the funding for my genital surgeries, and I was hoping that my consultant had been able to put my case forward. Whilst I waited for that to happen, I focussed on my recovery from my chest surgery and getting my body into good shape for the next phase.

I was really pleased with the changes that were happening which mainly featured the growth of facial hair. I had always wanted a beard and moustache, so to finally see the hair growing was fantastic. It was still early on in the process and the growth was very patchy but I knew that it could take years to grow a full beard, even for 'normal' men. I also knew that it would come through eventually, as I had always been pretty hairy before T, which was not ideal when I was female. I didn't really see many other changes; it was more noticeable to friends and family who didn't see me all the time. They would tell me that they could see changes in my jaw line and they also told me that my body was looking more masculine. However, I couldn't see those changes as they were subtle and, of course, as I saw myself every day the changes were not as obvious to me.

During this time, I started talking to a woman that I had met at Gay Pride some ten years before. She was the partner of one of my friends and, although we knew each other from a distance, we hadn't really talked properly. Over time, we had developed a really close friendship and I loved talking to her. She was a great listener and she was extremely interested in my journey. I learned that she was a therapeutic counsellor as well as having a full-time job and, because of her background in counselling, I instantly felt comfortable when we spoke.

As we got to know each other more closely, I started to feel an attraction toward her and I had a feeling that she felt the same way. This concerned me, as she was my friend's partner and I didn't want to cause any problems for them. From what I could see, they had a healthy and loving relationship and I didn't want to get in the way of that.

One day, I was invited to their house for drinks and dinner in the garden with some other friends. After dinner, she and I made desert together, a fruit crumble. I had never made a crumble before and asked her to show me how it was done. We drank wine in the kitchen, got a little 'sozzled' and then had, what we both now describe as, a Patrick Swayze and Demi Moore moment. Picture this, if you will - a large mixing bowl full of crumble topping, four hands in the mixing bowl covered in butter and flour, and those hands occasionally touching whilst binding the ingredients together. Well, let's just say that there were some sparks! All of this was going on whilst her partner and our friends were still in the garden. It didn't seem to matter to us that one of them could have come into the kitchen at any moment; it was exciting!

I stayed at their house that night and in the morning, after her partner (my friend) had left for work, I had an impulse to say to her, "don't go to work today, stay here with me". I didn't know what her reaction was going to be, but when I asked her to not go, she said that she would stay at home and that she would do some work later when I left. She didn't question why I had made that request, which made me think that she also felt that attraction and that we had both experienced the sparks flying above the mixing bowl the night before.

Later that morning, whilst having a bath, I asked her to come into the bathroom to chat. She did and, whilst I was in the bath, she sat on the toilet (seat closed) and we talked. It didn't feel strange to me at all - it felt as though we had been doing it for years. I could tell that she felt a little awkward, and rightly so; she was involved in a relationship with someone else, yet there she was talking to me whilst I was naked in the bath.

Later that morning, while we were downstairs together, I offered to give her a back massage. I know that this was very forward of me, but she seemed to like the idea and said yes. She sat on the floor whilst I sat on the sofa behind her, massaging her back; the atmosphere was electric! I could sense the anticipation in the air and I leaned down toward her and we kissed. At that time, I don't think either of us had considered what might lie ahead; it just felt right, and I hoped it would be the beginning of something rather beautiful.

We saw each other when we could, but things were difficult as she was still involved in another relationship. She had recently told me that she was unhappy in this relationship because it wasn't giving her what she needed. This was the first I had known about this, as they seemed so happy together. She said that her partner covered up the unhappiness when they were in social situations but that, behind closed doors, things were very different. This made me feel slightly better about the fact that I was seeing her behind her partner's back, because it meant that I wasn't intruding on a happy relationship.

Her name was Carla, and we continued to see each other. A while later, I received a call from her partner asking me if I was having a relationship with Carla; I lied and said no. I lied because, at that time Carla had not told her about us seeing each other and it wasn't my place to get involved. I had no idea at that time, whether Carla was intending to tell her, and I certainly didn't want to rock the boat.

Our relationship was getting stronger and stronger, and I knew how I felt about Carla. I knew that this was the woman with whom I wanted to spend the rest of my life. I had started to imagine how our life together could be and I could only imagine a life in which we were together. I knew that I wanted to ask her to marry me even though we hadn't been together for long. I started making plans about how, where and when I was going to ask her. I knew that she loved nature and walks and, considering where I lived and that I was surrounded by some beautiful countryside and woodland, I thought that would be a great place for it to happen.

Whilst out walking on my own one day, I came across a lovely area of woodland just down the road from my little hut. It was a beautiful sunny day and, as I was walking through the trees, it occurred to me that it would be the perfect location for a proposal. I thought about how I would ask Carla, and I decided that I would etch my proposal into the bark of a tree. This was going to take some time, and I would probably have to visit the tree more than once to do it. In light of my awful sense of direction and the fact that a lot of the trees looked the same, I marked the spot with two crosses. I was excited by the prospect of creating a cunning plan to entice Carla into the woods, but I knew that she loved walking and nature, so it wouldn't be too difficult.

I visited the tree over the next few weeks to finish the etching and also to plan the rest of the proposal. I certainly hadn't thought about buying an engagement ring and, at that time, I couldn't afford to buy one. I would need to find a temporary band that I could place on her finger if she said yes. I bought a length of red ribbon that I made into a band and I actually thought that it was quite romantic idea. I also bought some Prosecco and a couple of champagne glasses, so that we could make a toast- very presumptuous of me, I know. I wanted to have some music playing in the background, so I downloaded some soft, romantic music and connected an external speaker to my phone. I planned to put all the items into a rucksack and to say that we were going for a walk and that I had just packed some drinks and snacks. I was very excited, but I had no idea whether she would say yes.

We planned our next meeting, and we decided that she would visit me in my little hut in Sittingbourne. On the day, we chatted for a while and then I asked her if she would like to go for a country walk- I'm not really sure what would have happened if she had said no! We got ready to go for the walk and she asked me what was in the bag. I told her that it was drinks and snacks so that we could picnic somewhere if we wanted to.

It was a nice sunny day in June, and I remember the countryside surrounding us looking so beautiful. We walked up the lane which led to the woodland and, en route, we noticed a horse in a field, walking toward us. It walked right up to the fencing and stopped.

We walked over to meet the horse and spent some time stroking him - he was gorgeous. This gave me some breathing space as I was beginning to feel somewhat nervous! After a while, we continued up the lane toward the woods. I told Carla that I had previously walked there and I thought that she would really like it.

When we got into the thickest part of the woods, I felt a little internal panic as, although I had marked the spot with crosses, there were several woodland paths that could have sent us in the wrong direction. But I hadn't forgotten the way and I managed to find those trees. Carla hadn't noticed the crosses, as I had etched them quite high up on the two trees which stood side by side; they almost created an archway for us to walk through.

The tree carrying the etched proposal was just off the track, and so I had to tell her that I wanted to show her a particular tree. I am not sure what was going through her mind as she was being lured deeper into the woods.

I was now extremely nervous and I remember thinking, it's not too late to call it off and she would never know anything about it. As we approached the tree, we had to navigate the undergrowth to find a way through; I hadn't visited the tree for a little while and there had been a lot of new growth in that area. I held her hand whilst we walked between the trees and bushes trying not to get scratched to pieces. Finally, she said to me "where the hell are you taking me?" I just laughed and said she would know soon enough. Finally, we got to the tree and I said, "this is it". She had a somewhat bewildered look on her face, which made me giggle. The inscription was actually on the other side of the tree so that all she could see was a tree which looked a hell of a lot like all the other trees in the woods.

I suggested that we stop there for a drink and a rest and then opened up the rucksack to get the speaker and my phone so I could set it up to play some music. The look of bewilderment had deepened on her face and I could only imagine what she was thinking, but she just went along with it.

After a couple of minutes, I plucked up some courage and I asked her to come around to the other side of the tree with me as I wanted to show her something. Luckily, she followed me without asking any questions. I knelt on one knee on some rather prickly undergrowth, and pointed to the inscription on the tree. Carla looked up at the tree and read the inscription and, whilst she was doing that, I asked her if she would marry me.

She was visibly shocked, but I could see the wonderful smile that was developing on her face, as she said yes. I couldn't believe it; I was absolutely 'over the moon' and I felt I was the luckiest person alive. I went back into the rucksack and pulled out the red ribbon and placed it on her engagement finger. I told her that I hadn't bought an engagement ring yet, but she said she loved the ribbon and said it was so romantic.

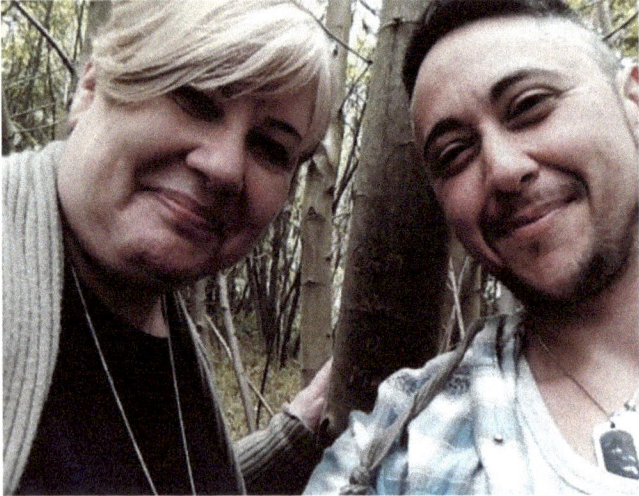

The proposal

We kissed and cuddled and just spent some time holding each other. I asked her if she would like a drink and pulled out the bottle of Prosecco and the Champagne glasses, so that we could drink a toast to celebrate. It was just perfect - I don't think it could have been any better. I remember her saying to me "you are a dark horse, aren't you?" I just smiled and said, "maybe I am".

When we had finished our Prosecco, we started the walk back to the hut. On the way, we walked past another couple who were also out walking. Suddenly Carla piped up and said "He just asked me to marry him". They smiled and congratulated us, and off we went, on our very merry way.

A few months passed and Carla and I were seeing each other as and when we could, as she lived near Heathrow and I was in Kent. We had talked about telling her partner that we were in a relationship, but had never really decided when this would happen.

One night, Carla called me and told me that she had told her partner that it was over between them and that she was in a relationship with me. Carla asked me for some time and breathing space because, although she knew it was the right thing to do, it was still extremely upsetting for both of them. I understood why she needed the time, although, I knew this would be difficult for me because I would miss her.

Although Carla had asked me for some time, she continued to call me most nights. She said that she wanted to check in on me to see how I was feeling but, also, I think she missed me. It was becoming increasingly more difficult to be apart. It wasn't long before we arranged to meet to spend some time together.

We continued to do this for a few weeks until Carla called me one day and asked if we could meet.

I remember that we went somewhere to eat and, on the way back she pulled into a petrol garage. She said that she needed to tell me something. I didn't like the sound of that and I clearly remember my heart pounding in my chest so hard that I thought it was going to burst through my skin.

She began to tell me that her partner had asked her if she would give their relationship another go. I was heart-broken, devastated and inconsolable. She explained that, in her heart, she knew that it wouldn't work, but that she had to at least try, after all, she did still love her. We sat for a while in the car and then eventually after a lot of tears, she drove me home to my parents' house.

I just couldn't get my head around it. Carla had agreed to marry me but she was going back to her ex. I think I understood her reasons, but at that time it just broke me! I contacted my very close friend and previous girlfriend and asked her if I could go and stay with her for a few days. She told me to come straight away and that I could spend as long as I liked with her.

When I arrived, we talked, she listened, I cried and then I didn't really stop crying for the whole time I was there. I vividly remember being in the bath, my body hunched over, in an almost foetal position with my head bowed low, just bawling my eyes out. My friend came into the bathroom just to try to console me, but she couldn't, so she just sat with me for a while.

I spent the evenings crying in her spare room and one night I snuck into her bed because I needed a cuddle. She was so good to me and just accepted that this was where I needed to be. I ended up spending a few days there before going back to my parents' house.

Carla continued to contact me because she knew how devastated I was and she told me how hard it was for her because she loved me so much. She just kept saying that she was trying to do the right thing. I was still so upset that whenever we spoke, I spent the majority of the call crying.

She told me that whether we were together, or just friends, she wanted to support me on my journey and that, if I wanted her there, she would come to any appointments with me. I was so grateful to her, not only for the support, but also because I would still see her, as I couldn't imagine my life without her in it.

Do you remember that I spoke earlier of the man I fell in love with who turned out to be gay? Well, it was whilst I had returned to stay with Mum and Dad, that I received the most awful news. I took a phone call from his husband who told me that he had died. He didn't know why but because it was a sudden death, there would need to be a post-mortem and coroner's report.

I was so shocked and really upset - he was only in his thirties. I knew that he was a drinker, probably an alcoholic, albeit a functioning alcoholic. When I first met him, he was quite a big guy and was certainly not lacking in confidence, as was I. He took it upon himself to lose weight and, with that, came a huge confidence boost.

Throughout our relationship I never suspected anything untoward, but it was after we split up and remained friends that it became evident that he suffered with Bulimia. He never talked about this or the alcoholism with me, but it became more apparent as time went on that he needed help.

We had fallen out for a period of time as he had quite an argumentative personality and it was whilst we were not talking, I learned of his untimely fate. I was so upset that we had not managed to forgive each other and that we had been on bad terms, not only because he didn't get to see me start my transitional journey, but because I loved him as a friend and I missed him terribly.

Carla was so supportive and was there for me 100% as she always was and I needed her then more than ever. It was so hard for me; as I needed her love, but all I could have was her friendship. Of course, she still loved me; it was just such an awful situation.

I had been asked to say some words about the relationship I had with him and I was so nervous that I thought I wouldn't be able to do it, but Carla came with me and it made me feel so much better-she was my rock on what was such an emotional day.

Chapter Ten - Decisions, Decisions and More Decisions

I finally received notification that my funding had been agreed and that I could proceed with my first consultation with one of the Uro-andrologists in the London Team. A Uro-andrologist is a specialist that is responsible for the diagnosis and treatment of any health issues related to the genito-urinary tract (relating to the genitals and urinary organs). This can include dealing with problems such as erectile dysfunction and penis reconstruction in natal males (born male). Some of these surgeons also have an interest in performing gender-confirming surgeries. Unfortunately, there are few consultants that have been trained to perform these surgeries as they are extremely complex micro-surgical procedures, and it can take a long time to reach the required level of expertise.

Carla and I attended the appointment together at St. Peters Andrology Centre in London on 8th June 2015. Carla was there to give me support, and we spent time with the consultant who talked to us about the detail of the options available.

Before this consultation I had spoken to some post-operative Trans guys to get a better sense of the possible outcomes of these surgeries. I wanted to find out whether there was a high percentage of people that had very little or no sensation following surgery. The feedback that I received was that a high percentage of people experienced a fairly good level of sensation, both tactile and sexual. I also discovered that the best surgical outcome with regard to sensation was experienced by the men who had opted for one particular technique which uses the forearm as the donor site. I am glad that I had spoken to these people, as it gave me some confidence and allowed me to put aside some of the worries I had experienced.

During the consultation, I was told about the two procedures that I could have; Metoidioplasty and Phalloplasty. I was told also, that there were variants within the Phallo procedure and this was going to make it even harder to choose what I wanted. Again, I felt that life was so unfair- why couldn't I just have been born 'normal'? By the way, when I use the term 'normal' I do so quite loosely because it just makes explanation easier. I don't, for one moment, think that there is such a thing as 'normal'. I suppose what I am trying to say is - why hadn't I been born a boy? Why should I or anyone else have to make such critical, life-changing decisions to become the person they should have been at birth.

The consultant told me to take as long as I needed to decide which would be the best option for me. I was conscious that I wanted to have made my decision by the end of the consultation because I didn't want to delay my progress any further. As I previously mentioned, there are different options to that particular surgery. The main difference being, from which part of the body the skin would be taken to create the penis. The consultant explained about the different donor sites which might be available and also about the pros and cons for each of those, and I will explain these below:

The Phallo procedure definitely has its positives, and those are: aesthetics, functionality and size. Unfortunately, sensation is very much a personal variant, as it is dependent on how well the person's nerves restore and connect after the procedure; this can take a few years, if they grow back at all. The level of sensation also varies and is dependent on the donor site used.

With the Meta procedure, the person would generally retain all sensation, unless there were complications. This procedure is also a lot less invasive and does not require as many surgeries. The drawbacks are the size that can be achieved, an issue not only aesthetically, but also 'in the bedroom'. The general appearance and the fact that the micro-penis would not clear the trouser fly, would make it difficult for the person to stand to urinate.

After listening to what the consultant had to say, my decision was definitely swaying towards Radial Forearm Phalloplasty (RAP), however, one of the drawbacks with RAP, is that the donor site would be completely visible and there would be a large area of scarring, noticeable to others. Human beings are inquisitive creatures and this should definitely be a consideration when deciding about whether to have this particular procedure. There would always be the option of having that area tattooed once significant healing has taken place, but not before two years. This would mean that the individual may have to cover their forearm until such a time as they can get it tattooed.

Other considerations are aesthetics and functionality over sensation. Appearance and functionality were hugely important to me, but I also wanted to feel tactile and sexual sensation. What would be the point of having a penis that looked good and performed well and then potentially not being able to feel anything? I wanted to be able to feel closest to what a 'normal' man would feel.

The consultant told me that if I went for RAP, they would create the penis in the first operation, but that I would have to undergo two further surgeries, to complete the rest of the work to make everything look right and make it functional. He told me that, in some countries, the creation of the penis (phallus) and all the other procedures that are done to make it functional, can be done in one operation, but that in the UK, the surgeons do it in separate stages to allow the body enough time to adjust and heal.

Nearing the end of the consultation, after having talked about all the options and having considered the pros and cons of each of them, I had decided that I wanted to have the procedure known as Radial Arm Phalloplasty (RAP)

Once I had made the decision, the surgeon was then able to tell me more about what was involved in that specific surgical procedure. Before we went any further, he asked to see my forearm and more particularly, my non-dominant arm. The surgeons will always try to use the non-dominant arm in case there are any issues after the surgery and also, recovery is easier if the dominant arm is not used. He wanted to check the blood flow to this arm and hand and, in order to do this, he used a method called the Allen Test. He explained that he would apply pressure to the radial and ulnar arteries in my wrist for several seconds to stop the blood flow to my hand. When the pressure is released, the ulnar artery should go pink, showing that there is adequate blood flow to the hand and arm. If the results are poor, they would usually follow on by doing a Doppler vascular scan. This scan allows the surgeon to take a measurement of the blood vessels. If they measure more than 2mm in diameter, they can normally proceed, and use the forearm as the donor site.

He also wanted to see how hairy my arms were, especially the underneath of my forearms because that area would be used in the creation of my urethra. I was pleased to hear that I had a good blood-flow and that he didn't feel I needed to have any laser hair removal. Laser hair-removal can take up to a year and involves several sessions which can be quite painful and this would inevitably, delay my surgery.

Although Carla was with me during the consultation, she remained quiet, other than to ask a few questions. I would occasionally look at her, almost hoping that she would help me to make this huge decision. She could see by my facial expression, that I was looking to her for guidance but she said, simply "this has to be your decision"

The consultant told me that the first surgery is extremely complex and takes 8-10 hours to perform and that I would need to be in hospital for at least 7 days afterwards. The lengthy hospital stay is needed as there are several surgical sites involved that need specialist care, and the hospital team is trained to care for patients after this type of procedure. Finally, the consultant told me that there was a waiting list for surgery, but that he would get me in as soon as he could.

Below, I will explain what each of the stages of RAP involves. The order in which these happen is generally similar, however this can depend on the surgeon who is performing the procedure and also how the individual heals after each stage. The recommended time frame between each stage is three months, as this allows for significant healing to take place:

This is a diagram of the stages of phalloplasty using different areas of the body as the donor site. Credit to St. Peters Andrology Centre London and Mr Nim Christopher MPHIL FRCS (UROL), Consultant Uroandrologist for the images.

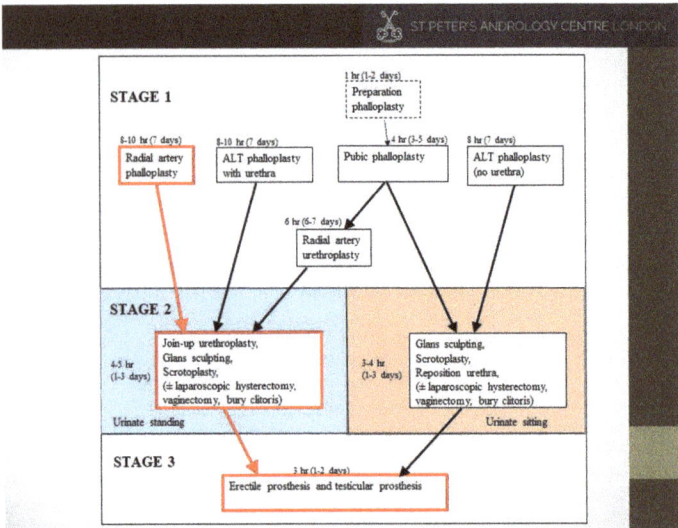

The procedure I chose is highlighted in red

Stage One: This involves the formation of a penis by taking skin and fat from the radial forearm. This donor site is supposed to have the best results when it comes to sensation because the surgeon would be able to harvest one of the main arteries in the forearm and attach it to the new penis. Unfortunately, in other phalloplasty procedures, this is generally not possible.

The surgeon takes two rectangular shaped pieces of skin and fat from the forearm, one large and one smaller in width, but longer. The larger piece of skin consists of most of the top side of the lower forearm. The smaller piece is taken from the underneath of the forearm and this is the part that is used to make the urethra. A nerve is taken from the donor site to try to provide a better outcome with regard to sensation; an artery is also taken to preserve the blood flow.

Once the skin and fat have been taken from the forearm, a thinner layer of skin and fat is taken from another area of the body to form a full-thickness skin graft. The most commonly used area for the graft to be taken from is the buttocks. This skin is taken from just underneath the buttocks and is generally the best area with the right amount of fat and, because of where it is, it will be well hidden.

The donor skin, including the nerve and the artery are then rolled up into a sausage shape to form the phallus, with the inside of the forearm being used to create a tube (the urethra). The reason that the inner part of the arm is used for the urethra is that this part of the arm is less hairy; hair in the urethra could cause problems later on.

Once the phallus has been created, two holes are made, one in the groin area and one in the pubic area, and this is where the phallus, the nerve and the artery are connected to the body. The new urethra is then redirected to a hole that is made at the base of the phallus; this enables the individual to flush the urethra to keep it open and clean. However, the new urethra cannot be used for urination until Stage Two.

Below are some pictures showing the stages of surgery involved during the phalloplasty procedure.

Credit St. Peters Andrology Centre London and Mr Nim Christopher MPHIL FRCS (UROL), Consultant Uroandrologist

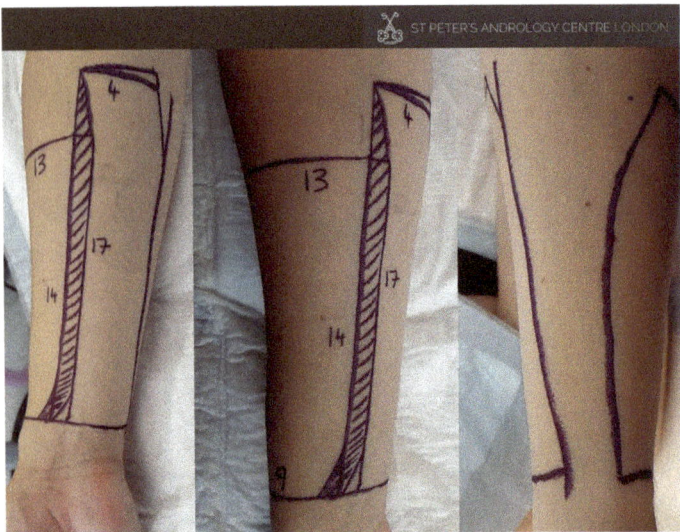

The drawings on the arms with measurements,
in preparation for the creation of the phallus

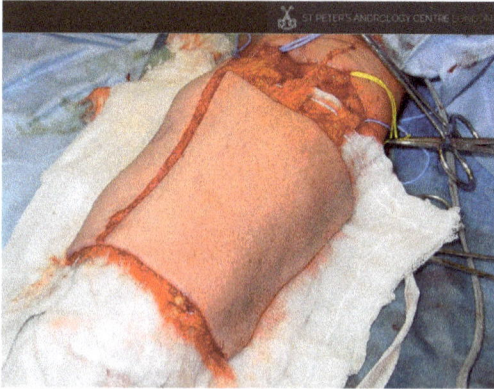

Once the flap has been created, it is elevated in preparation
for removal from the forearm;
the cephalic vein and nerves are attached

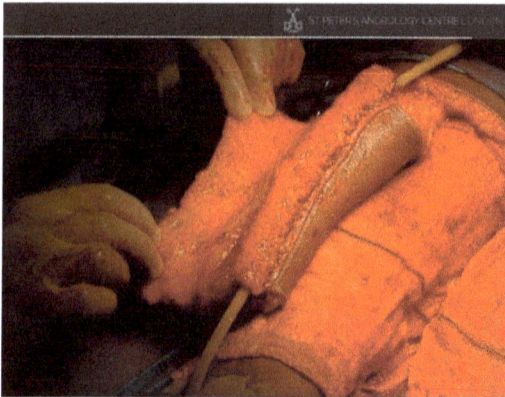

Once the flap has been removed, it is then rolled into a
sausage shape with a hollow centre. A stent is placed through
the centre to maintain patency (to keep open) to allow for
post-operative flushing. The phallus has to be flushed to
keep it clean, otherwise it has a tendency to smell.
The reason for the hollow centre is to prepare for the
urethral extension and hook-up (Stage Two), which will
allow the patient to void (urinate) through the phallus.

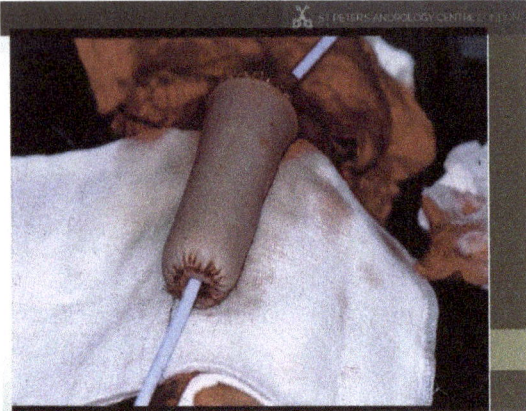

This image shows the phallo after it has been rolled up and stitched together with the stent inside.

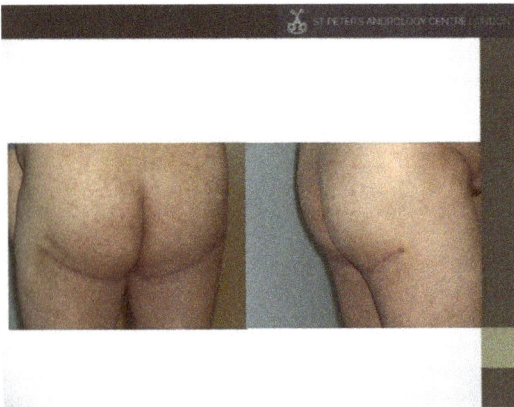

This image shows where skin and fat are taken from underneath
the buttocks to create a full-thickness graft,
which replaces the skin and fat taken from the forearm.
The wounds are closed with staples - up to 80 are used.
This is an ideal area to take the graft from, as the wound sits
nicely underneath the buttock cheeks and is therefore well
hidden. The other benefit of using this area is that it gives the
patient a nice bum-tuck at the same time.

Stage Two: This involves hooking up the urethra, a scrotoplasty, a total hysterectomy and glans sculpting. The urethra is redirected from the bladder to the end of the phallus. Once this has been completed, the original urethra is then closed as it no longer has a use. At this stage, if the individual has chosen to have a vaginectomy (a procedure that removes part, or all, of the vagina) this will also be done. Some individuals choose not to have this done as they want to retain that part for sexual purposes and this would mean that they would still be able to have penetrative sex. Also, at this stage, the individual will undergo a total abdominal hysterectomy and bilateral salpingo-oophorectomy (the surgical removal of the ovaries)

The genital area is then prepared for scrotoplasty, the creation of the scrotum. One common method used is to create the scrotal sack by moving the skin from the labia to create a sack. The individual would also have been given the choice to either bury the clitoris underneath the skin of the sack, or to leave it where it is and not bury it. Some individuals choose to leave it where it is and not bury it, as they don't mind how it will look; it can also be hard to locate underneath the sack. If the surgeon is burying the clitoris, one of its two nerves is harvested to connect to the base of the phallus so that there is more chance of sexual sensation. Removing one of the nerves doesn't seem to affect the sensation to the clitoris as it can function pretty well with only one.

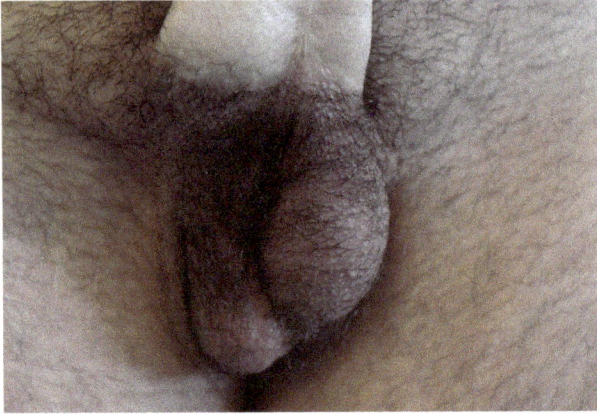

Above is a picture of my Scrotoplasty with testicular implants 'in situ'. I was never much good at documenting my journey with photos and I only managed to get a few images, so this photo is a recent one

The last part of this procedure is called glans sculpting, which is when the head of the penis is created. This is done by removing a strip of skin from the tip of the phallus which is then folded underneath itself to create what looks like a hem. For aesthetic reasons, a small skin graft is taken from either the abdomen or the hip; this makes the phallus look more realistic and changes it from having a sausage-like appearance, to that of a real penis.

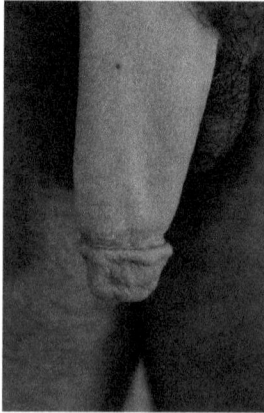

Above is a picture of my Glans sculpting/Glansplasty-
also a recent picture

Stage Three: This involves the placing of testicular implants
(balls) made from silicone, and an erectile device. If the
individual wants to experience an erection, they would
need to have the device placed inside the phallus. There are
different types available, and the individual would need to
have chosen which one would best suit them. One of these
devices is a malleable rod which enables the individual
to bend the phallus into the right position for penetration.
In this case, the individual would be given two silicone
implants as balls. Another option is to have a cylinder
placed into the phallus; this would enable the individual to
achieve an erection by squeezing a pump to be located in
the other side of the testicular sack, so there would be only
one ball and one pump. The pump is connected to a
reservoir filled with saline that is placed into the individual's
abdomen. To achieve an erection, the individual would
need to squeeze the pump in the scrotum, allowing the
saline to be drawn down from the reservoir and into the

cylinder in the phallus, thus making it hard. Incidentally, natal born males with erectile dysfunction, can also have this procedure carried out, to allow them to achieve an erection. Having finished with the pump, the saline is then returned to the reservoir by squeezing another part of the pump mechanism.

Penile prosthesis

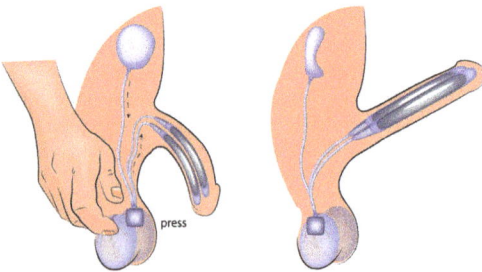

This image shows an example of an erectile device and how it works. It also shows the placement of the device inside the phallus.

This is not the exact implant that was used in my procedure but it gives an idea of where everything sits, and its function.

This particular image was taken from a website that provides penile prostheses for natal males who require such devices for various reasons. I found it difficult to find an image that represented the placement of the prosthesis in a Transgender FTM patient, so please note that the pump site in this example is not correct as, for the specific purpose, it would have to be placed inside one of the empty testicular sacks.

As you will see, the pump which is shown next to the hand, sits between the testicles on a natal male. However, it would be sited inside either the right or left testicular sack on an FTM Transgender patient.

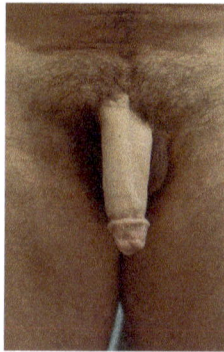

This is an image showing my phallus in its flaccid state before inflation using the pump.

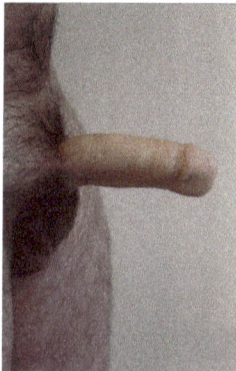

This is an image showing my phallus in its erect state after inflation using the pump.

The RAP procedure requires the individual to have three to four operations, not including any potential complications that may require surgical revisions. Some of the complications that can occur are infections or haematomas (localised bleeding outside of the blood vessels that can occur due to surgery or trauma). Haematomas can be extremely painful, especially in that part of the body. In most cases these would be absorbed back into the blood stream over a period of time. In some cases, however, surgical intervention may be required to evacuate the blood from that area. If the patient were to become infected, they would need to take antibiotics either orally or intravenously, through a drip. If left untreated, a patient could end up with sepsis, a potentially life-threatening condition caused by the body's response to an infection. There are many other complications, too many to mention here, that can also hinder an individual's recovery.

For your information, below is a diagram of all of the different surgical routes dependent on the chosen donor site.

By the end of the consultation, my head was swimming because of all the information I had been given. It was overwhelming, but I also felt really happy. This surgery was going to give me the new body I so desperately desired.

On the way home, Carla and I talked about the consultation and about my thoughts and feelings. As always, she listened intently. She told me that she'd had no idea how complicated it all would be and that it was going to take a huge toll on me, both mentally and physically. I agreed, but I just had to do this, I had no choice.

Chapter Eleven - It's Actually Happening!

A few weeks passed and Carla and I were still in regular contact. One day she called me and said that she couldn't continue trying to reconcile things with her ex. She loved me and couldn't continue to live a lie. Nothing had changed in her former relationship and she told me that her ex probably didn't want us to be together and that's why she suggested for them to try again. I didn't care about the reason, I was just 'over the moon' and spent the time until our next meeting feeling truly happy and content.

I couldn't believe that she wanted to be with me knowing that I intended to change my body forever. Carla had been in heterosexual relationships before and has two children, but she was never happy with men, and so came out as Lesbian.

All I could hope for was that she wouldn't change her mind later on when she saw how much my body was changing. One thing I did know was that I was still the same person, and that it was just my shell that was changing. I had to believe that this would be the reason that we would be together and I would still be the person that she fell in love with.

I received a copy of the report from the consultant which had also been sent to my GP. In the report, the consultant explained that I would be undergoing RAP, a testicular prosthesis, a laparoscopic (keyhole) hysterectomy, a vaginectomy, join-up urethroplasty (redirection of the urethra), a burying of the clitoris, glans sculpting (creation of the head of the penis) and penile prosthesis (erectile device). He advised that I was ready for surgery and that I would receive a date for Stage One as soon as was practicable. Oh my, suddenly it was all so real and was actually happening!

After having been at my parents' house for a while, I went back to my little hut in Kent, but I knew that the time was fast approaching for me to give notice to my lovely landlady. Because we had already talked about my transition, I knew that this wouldn't be a hard conversation to have. I wanted to be completely honest with her as we had built such a lovely friendship. I knew that I would miss her terribly and I also knew that she would miss having me around. I was also going to miss my little hut and its beautiful surroundings.

One day, whilst having coffee with her, I told her that I had been listed for surgery and that I would have to give my notice. I wasn't able to tell her when this would happen as I was yet to receive my date, but I wanted her to be prepared for the time when I would need to move out. She had already told me that she would need to get another lodger as the rent helped her to pay for some of the maintenance on her house and land. She said that she would be so sad to see me go, but that she completely understood. I felt a sense of relief after telling her, because it was one thing on a long list of things I needed to do to prepare for my surgery.

As time marched on, I was becoming a little impatient as I hadn't heard anything about my appointment for Stage One, although because I knew that people could sometimes wait over a year for surgery, I hadn't expected to receive a date before the end of 2015. Having said that, I still needed to make preparations and give notice at my work, of the dates I would be on leave, and I just needed a focus.

In August, to my surprise, I received a phone call from the surgical co-ordinator at St. Peters Andrology Centre. He asked me if I was flexible with my admission date for Stage One because there had been a cancellation and a slot had become available on 27th October 2015 at the hospital of St. John and St. Elizabeth in London. I remember freezing for a brief moment as I wasn't expecting that to happen. I managed to gather myself together and said "yes, I'll take it". We spoke a little about what would happen on the day of my admission, but he told me that he would be sending me some information that I would need to read, and some forms that I would need to complete and send back to him.

When the call ended, my thoughts were all over place. I was excited, nervous and scared, all at the same time. Although I had been through top surgery already, this was a much bigger operation and would involve a lot more planning. I remember thinking, "ok, what the hell do I do now? Who do I need to call? What do I need to get ready? I have always been a very practical person and once I have been given a date or a time-frame to do something, I just get on with it; I am not one to procrastinate.

I had phone calls to make to friends and family. Not only did I want them to share in my excitement, I also needed some moral support and someone to tell me 'it's all going to be ok'. I knew that whomever I called, be it Mum, Dad, Carla or any one of my friends, I would get that reassurance I so desperately needed.

I was so lucky to have a support network, as not everyone is this fortunate. Many people have to face going through transition alone because their family and friends do not accept them for who they are, and I cannot imagine how hard that must be. This is why support groups are invaluable, as they almost provide an adopted family for those people.

When I spoke to Mum, I could hear the excitement and anticipation in her voice. She told me that she was scared, not only for me, but also for herself. She knew exactly what these surgeries entailed because we had talked about the detail, so she had every right to be worried.

I set about planning and writing lists- I do love a good list! I didn't know what I would need to take to hospital with me. Luckily, I had joined some Facebook groups that support individuals struggling with their identity and one group, in particular, was specifically set up to support people who are going through Phalloplasty surgeries. This group was my go-to place when I had any questions about surgery. I posted on the group regularly to ask questions about what I should expect before, during and after surgery, and I found that I always received a great response. Some responses came from people that had been through these procedures, but I also received responses from people who hadn't yet been through them. The responses varied a little because there were so many different procedures and, also, outcomes to those procedures. This group provided a safe place for me to ask anything I wanted.

I posted on the group to ask about preparation for Stage One and, more specifically, about what I would need to take to hospital with me. Once again, I received the answers I needed and I was provided with lists that other people had used.

Now that I had a date for surgery, the next thing I needed to do was to notify my manager at work. I arranged to have a meeting with her during work time. At that meeting, I told her about the date for surgery and the estimated time off that I would need for recovery, but I could only give an approximate recovery time based on other people's experiences. I explained some of the procedures to her and, as always, she was very supportive, showing so much care and interest.

I told her about how they would create my willy and from where they would take the skin. We laughed when I said that she would actually be able to touch my buttocks after surgery because it would be on my arm.

Because I didn't know how long my recovery would take following the Stage One process, and how long a delay there would be before I had Stages Two and Three, I said that I may need to hand in my notice. I explained that the process could go on for a couple of years, dependent on waiting lists, surgery time and recovery time. She told me that she didn't want me to leave and that she would keep my job open for me so that I could return after everything was complete. She explained that I wouldn't be paid for this time as it would have to be designated as sick-leave. I was so grateful for this offer, as it meant I would have a job to return to, once it was all over.

Although there was going to be a huge financial impact to this, I had to make sure I had the time I needed to recover from each stage. Some people have to go back to work in between stages as they need to keep earning, but because I was fortunate enough to be able to stay with my parents, I didn't have to worry about paying rent and bills etc.

At the end of the meeting, we agreed a leaving date and then she gave me a big hug and told me how brave I was to put myself through all of this. I told her that, to me, it's wasn't about bravery, it was just something I had to do.

I also spoke to Carla and she offered to take me to hospital on the day of my admission and said that she would spend as much time there with me as her work permitted. I was so grateful to have the person I loved by my side and I knew that it would really help me to cope.

Chapter Twelve - It's a Boy!

Over the next couple of months, I concentrated on focussing my mind, trying to make sure that I was as emotionally ready as I could be. This was difficult because, really, I had no idea of what was to come. I knew what to expect from the physical aspects of the surgery, but I knew nothing of the emotional realities. All I knew was that this was going to be one hell of a ride!

A week before I was due to be admitted, I had an appointment at the hospital for pre-op tests including; blood tests, blood-pressure and temperature checks, and swabs to check for MRSA, all very similar to what was done before my chest surgery. Once again, I was given a clean bill of health and was told that, provided that the swabs were negative and my bloods were ok, I would be admitted as planned.

The time seemed to fly and before I knew it, October 27th 2015 had arrived. I was so excited and, naturally, also very scared, but I had my love by my side which made things so much better. Carla had always shown me compassion and understanding, and this time was no different.

On the way to the hospital, we talked but some of the journey was spent in complete silence. I was trying my best to combat my nerves, but I found this really difficult. I knew that Carla sensed this and left me to my own thoughts and that was exactly what I needed at that time. My admission to the hospital was actually the night before the surgery. The London team requires the patient to be in the hospital the night before their scheduled surgery time, as they begin their surgeries very early in the morning.

Carla spent most of the evening with me and we passed the time by get me settled into my room, unpacking my bag and familiarising ourselves with the room. It was a very nice private room, and it was spacious, with lots of room for visitors. There was a flat-screen TV on the wall with a remote-control, something for which I was very grateful, given my history of not sleeping well after anaesthesia.

My room was on a floor with patients having many different procedures, including those who were having transition surgery. To fill in some time, we decided to walk around the ward and Carla noticed that the door of one of the rooms was open. She became inquisitive, as she saw that the man in the room had his arm raised and in a sling. She asked me if this was what I would have to do after surgery. I said that it looked like he had just had the Stage One procedure and that his arm might be in the sling to keep the hand from swelling. We had made an assumption that he was Trans - he looked like an ordinary man with his arm in a sling so, for all we knew, he could have broken it.

Being the friendly person that she is, Carla said to me, "he's on his own; he might appreciate some friendly faces, shall we go in and say hello?" I am more reserved and can be shy when meeting new people, so I was a little hesitant but I did agree. We knocked on the open door and asked if it was okay for us to go in. He said "of course, you are very welcome" Carla is not shy and she said "please forgive us if we have made the wrong assumption, but have you had transition surgery?" He told us not to worry and that, yes, he had just been through Stage One.

I was so pleased that we had gone into his room - he was so lovely. He talked me through what was going to happen to me and what to expect after the surgery. It was great to talk to someone, in the flesh, who had just had the procedure I was about to have.

In the morning, I was visited by the consultant, Mr Nim Christopher, who I had seen at St Peters Andrology Centre. He had such a happy and pleasant demeanour, which I found very comforting. He talked to me about what he and the team would be doing and asked me if I understood everything. He said that I was 2nd on his list because there was one patient going before me who had an underlying health condition and those patients always take priority.

Shortly after this, the anaesthetist visited me and, as with my previous surgery (double mastectomy), he asked me a series of health-related questions and also if I was allergic to anything. I told him of my concerns about feeling sick after surgery and he said not to worry, he would make sure that I had an anti-sickness drug throughout, and after the surgery.

The nursing team visited me a few times to give me various things in preparation for surgery. I was, again, given surgical stockings to help prevent blood clots forming due to post-surgery inactivity. I was also given a surgical gown and some anti-bacterial wash, and was asked to shower approximately an hour before surgery and to wash thoroughly with the anti-bacterial wash. Wow, this was getting real, no turning back now!

Anticipating my surgery, I felt anxious, but so excited at the prospect of waking afterward with a 'sausage' between my legs. This was going to be a moment I would remember for the rest of my life!

I didn't have to wait long before a team of people came to whisk me away to theatre. Carla was able to walk with me to the theatre doors where we were able to say our goodbyes. This was really quite emotional and, although not wishing to be morbid, I recognised that this operation could take ten hours and, like any surgery, there were always risks. Carla smiled at me, kissed me on the cheek and said "see you on the other side"

I remember entering the anaesthesia room. The lights were so bright and everything was pristine and clinical looking. The anaesthetic team was so kind and caring, and they all made me feel less nervous by talking to me and making things as light-hearted as possible. I was given a nice pre-med which worked quickly and, after placing a cannula in my hand, they told me they would be injecting the anaesthetic and that I was to count down from ten. I remember asking the team what that funny smell was but that was it- lights out.

When I awoke in the recovery room, it seemed as if I had only been out for a few minutes. I don't remember feeling much pain; however, I did feel sick and asked the nurse for some more anti-sickness drug. I spent some time in the recovery room as my blood pressure was quite low. Generally, my blood pressure is on the lower side of normal, but it had dropped much more significantly. Once they had managed to stabilise it a little, I was moved back to my room. Carla was waiting for me there and she had been in the hospital the entire time I was in surgery. She told me that she had been worried because I was gone for a longer period of time than was expected. The nurse explained that they had been monitoring my blood pressure as it had dropped quite low. Carla was thrilled to see me and kissed me and gave me a gentle hug. She had to be careful as my donor arm was up in a sling at a 90-degree angle to stop my hand swelling.

I was awake, but not very lucid as I had been anaesthetised for so long. I do remember talking to her, and the nurses and doctors who were in and out of my room, but I don't remember much of what was said. I do know, though, that I had a smile on my face and I was a happy boy.

Throughout the rest of the evening, I had many visits from the nursing team. They were checking my blood-pressure regularly and also my other vital signs, oxygen levels and temperature. My blood-pressure was slowly starting to rise, but I was told that I needed to drink plenty of fluids to help with this. My oxygen saturation was good and my temperature was normal. I was on a drip to maintain my fluid balance and I had a morphine pump, which I could use to administer small doses, as and when I needed them. I remember very vividly, the many tubes and wires that were going into my body.

Even though my surgery was funded by the NHS, I was in a private hospital which had no set visiting hours, and this meant that Carla could stay for as long as she wanted. It was comforting to know that she was there, even if I wasn't particularly lucid.

During that evening, I also had a visit from Mum and Dad and it was so lovely to see them. As the evening went on, I had another visit from a nurse and, as well as checking my vital signs, she needed to perform a Doppler test on my sausage to check for blood flow. This is to make sure that there was a pulse and that everything looked ok. They were also checking to make sure that there was no excessive oozing or bleeding. This was the first time that I would see my new willy. The only problem was, I was flat on my back and had to get Carla to take a picture of it for me.

It was a surreal moment for me because, as I lay there, Mum, Dad and Carla were at the foot of my bed looking at my sausage. This is something I never would have imagined happening! I remember the nurse saying "That's a big one" and, of course, we all burst out laughing.

The nurse did the Doppler test by putting a probe against a certain point in the phallus and we could all hear the beating. It was like having a baby scan and I remember saying "it's a boy!" There is always a risk of the phallus not getting the blood flow, so it was great to hear that beat.

During the surgery, a catheter had been placed directly into my bladder through my existing urethra and the reason for this is so that I would not have to get out of bed to pee for at least three days. This catheter would then be removed and I would be left with a stent in my phallus until the day of discharge. The stent is only placed there to keep the tunnel in my phallus open and clear. After Stage One, I still had to sit down to pee, as I was yet to have the urethra lengthened, re-routed and hooked up and this would all be done at Stage Two.

Over the course of all my operations I came to realise that catheters are the work of the devil! They caused more problems for me than the actual surgical sites themselves. I later found out that catheter problems are quite common and a lot of people end up with them blocking or causing horrendous bladder spasms.

Over the next few days, Carla visited as much as she could and I also had visits from friends. I enjoyed this so much and it definitely helped to keep me occupied. I have never been very good at doing nothing and it was even harder in hospital, because this inactivity was medically imposed on me, giving me no choice. Luckily, I was so exhausted for most of the time, that I didn't really mind doing nothing. The time passed quickly and, before I knew it, the physio team was there, preparing me for my first attempt at standing up. Carla and her daughter were with me that day, so they were there to see me stand up for the first time.

The physio team warned me that, as with my previous surgery, my blood pressure would probably drop as I had been lying down for three days and this is exactly what happened. They told me to try to get myself into a sitting position first, using the side of the bed as an aid. This was a struggle because, as there were so many areas of my body that had been operated on, it was really quite painful. I did manage it in the end, but it took several attempts.

I remained sitting for a few minutes to allow my blood-pressure to normalise. Once I felt ready, and with the help of the team, I managed to stand. I only managed it for a brief moment though, because I felt as if I was going to pass out, so I had to sit down again on the edge of the bed. Both Carla and her daughter were obviously concerned and said afterwards that they could almost see the life draining out of my face because I went so pale. I have to say that it wasn't a pleasant experience! The team decided that they would let me lay down again and that we would try again the next day. I was relieved as I felt worn out, and for the remainder of the day I just rested and chatted with Carla and her daughter.

Mr Christopher also visited me on this day so he could check my phallus and all the other surgical sites. He was also very pleased with my progress and asked me about my pain level. I told him that the main area causing me pain was my buttocks and, also, that the catheters were very uncomfortable. He said that it is very common to experience this with the catheters, especially the one in the bladder as it rests against the bladder wall and causes the bladder to spasm. All in all, he said he was pleased with all the surgical sites and that I should be discharged according to the original plan.

On the next day, my attempt at standing was better and I managed to stand up with the help of the physios. I even managed to walk to the visitors' chair and, once there, they helped lower me into it so that I could sit and rest. They wanted me to spend a couple of hours out of bed in the chair, to allow my body to become used to sitting upright, also helping my blood pressure to remain stable. Sitting was so painful, as I had nearly eighty staples below my buttocks, which was the area from where the graft had been taken for my forearm. As well as having a catheter in my bladder, the surgical team had placed another one in my phallus. The phallus catheter is used to keep the new urethra open and ready for when the time came to flush it. Both of these catheters made sitting very uncomfortable.

I stayed in the chair for about an hour before calling a nurse to ask for help to get back into bed. The nurse asked me to try to stay for a while longer because it is more beneficial to recovery than lying down all the time. Reluctantly, I agreed and managed another hour.

Carla was continuing to visit me in the hospital as often as she could and she helped me to move around my room, also accompanying me on short walks along the corridors. She also had to help me shower as I was still very incapacitated and it took all my strength just to walk to the wet room, a few doors down.

When she helped me with my first shower, she had to help with everything, including undressing, and this was the first time she had seen me naked. I could see by her face that something was wrong and deep down, I thought I knew what the problem might be. I said to her "is this (my willy) going to be a problem?" She said that seeing me naked in front of her brought everything into perspective. We talked a little about what she was feeling and she said that seeing me like that was really difficult, because I looked like a man!

Of course, I did look like a man, and that was the whole point of all of this! What she meant was, seeing me like that had brought home the reality of her being in a relationship with a man, something she had never thought would happen again. I tried to understand how she was feeling but, in that moment, I felt hurt. After talking some more, she said that if I were any other man, she wouldn't even entertain a relationship, but because it was me and she loved me, it wasn't going to be a deal breaker; I was so relieved!

Over the next few days, my recovery progressed well and the nursing and physio teams were very happy with how I was doing. Although it was still very painful, I was able to spend more and more time out of bed. By the end of the week, I was definitely ready to go home as I was starting to become a little stir crazy.

When the time came for my discharge, I was already packed and couldn't wait to get going. My going home outfit was a very loose pair of jogging bottoms and a comfy jumper. My willy had to be padded and kept up at a 45-degree angle towards my stomach which allows for healing underneath. The loose jogging bottoms were a must, as I am sure you can imagine the looks one might get walking around with one's willy sticking out at such an angle!

On the morning of my discharge, the stent was removed from my phallus and then, once I had seen the discharge nurse and she had all my medications ready, I was free to go. I was so pleased to get out of there but I was not really looking forward to the hour-long journey home. I was given some Oramorph® (oral morphine) to take before I left to make the journey a little more comfortable. Carla wheeled me out of my room and to the car which she had already parked close to the exit. It was so good to get some fresh air and be out of my room.

We made it back to Mum's and Dad's house in good time but it was a very uncomfortable journey, as I felt every bump and pothole in the road.

Chapter Thirteen - Bobbing Along

Once at Mum's and Dad's house, I was settled into my little annexe room and I rested for the afternoon. I was so lucky to have been able to recuperate there as I had my own bedroom with an adjoining shower room and toilet, which made everything so much easier for me. I also received the raised toilet seat that a friend had kindly posted to me and what a God-send that was! It was still uncomfortable to sit on the toilet, but it was so much better with the padded seat.

My discharge plan had been already sent to my GP and it included dressing changes, wound care and staple removal. All of these things were to be provided by a district nurse who would visit me at home. I spoke to the district nursing team and we arranged an appointment for the first dressing change on my arm, to take place one week after discharge. The dressing was to be left in place until then to cause minimal disturbance to the wound and, when I showered, I had to put a plastic bag over my arm to keep the dressing dry.

The staples in my buttocks were also due to be removed and they would be done at the same time as the dressing change. I really wasn't looking forward to having them removed as I had heard that this could be rather painful. I looked on the Internet to see if I could find any numbing cream which might help. The problem was that those creams couldn't be used on open wounds and, as some of the incision line was still open, I wouldn't be able to use the cream.

The day came for my staple removal and dressing change and, although I was excited about seeing how my arm was healing, I was not looking forward to the staples coming out. I don't have a high pain threshold, so this was not going to be easy for me.

Carla and Mum were in the room with me for moral support. When the nurse arrived, she said that she was concerned about what she had been asked to do. She had not seen any Transgender patients before and had not been given any training on the post-surgical requirements. She was so concerned, that she actually made a call to the St. John and St. Elizabeth hospital to ask what she was required to do. They told her to follow the directions on the post-op care plan, and to treat the wound like any other wound and dress it according to their instructions. She said was not overly concerned about the staple removal because this was straightforward.

After she had finished talking to the hospital, we began to talk about the lack of awareness in the medical profession about gender-confirming surgeries. She told us that she certainly hadn't received any training on aftercare, and hadn't known what to expect.

I explained my surgery to her, and she said that it was amazing and how brave I was. She told me that for any future district nurse appointments, I should ask for her so that there would be some continuity and she would know how the wounds were healing from one appointment to the next. I agreed that this would definitely be the best thing.

The first thing she did was take off all the dressings on my donor arm. It felt so nice when they were off and to have air on my skin. She was very impressed with the graft and said that it was healing well. I am a little squeamish, and this was only the second time that I had seen the graft after surgery. When I looked at my arm, I actually felt okay and I was interested to see how it was doing. Once she was happy with how things looked, she redressed it.

The next surgical site she needed to check was my pubic area, where my phallus had been attached. She removed the padding and checked the wound and, again, said that it looked really good and was healing well. She was absolutely amazed by the work of the surgeon! She redressed that area and, again, padded it up to the 45-degree angle again. The phallus has to be kept at that angle for three weeks post-surgery.

Next came the staple removal, the part that I was most dreading! I was asked to lie on my front so that the nurse could get to the staples easily, and, at least I was lying down, because this bit really hurt! Some of the staples had become embedded in my skin and she had a really tough time getting them out, having to dig into my skin with the staple remover to try to ease them away from the wound. I had to ask her to stop on more than one occasion. Eventually, she managed to get them all out. There were a couple of areas that were still a little bit open but, overall, the wound had sealed very well.

At my first wound review on the 4th November 2015, the nurse practitioner said that the phallus was healing well and that it was nice and warm, a sign of good blood flow; also, there was no sign of infection. She also said that there was a lot of superficial bruising to my phallus, the base of the phallus and my upper thighs, but told me not to worry, as this would not last. There were some areas of blistering on my arm but it was healing, and the graft had taken well. The nurse redressed my arm with Mepitel, a very specific type of dressing used for this purpose.

I was given a Speedi Cath (a catheter that is used to flush the urethra), and was told that once the swelling and bruising had reduced, I could gently pass this down the urethra so that it remained patent (open). I was then shown how to flush the urethra with saline and was advised to do this daily. To flush the phallus, I was given a syringe and told to fill it with warm water and then to direct it into the hole that was the old urethra. Once it was in the hole, I had to slowly syringe the water through until it came out of the end of the phallus.

Over the course of the next couple of months, I had a couple more bandage changes which were done by the district nurse but, between nurse visits, I was advised to let some air get to the graft. I was also asked to start bathing my arm in salty water.

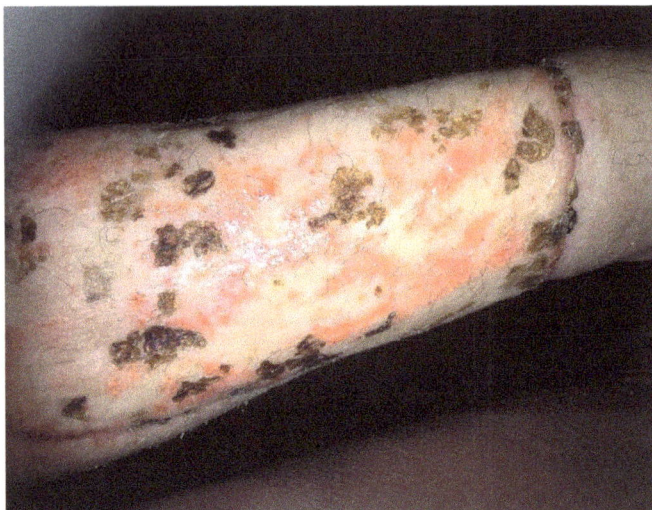

This picture shows my arm at the stage where most of the healing has taken place. There were just a few areas of scabbing that needed to come off.

Now that I was able to get the arm wet, I could also shower without the plastic bag. I had begun to bath my arm regularly, and both Mum and Carla learned how to redress my arm so that I wouldn't need to have a nurse do it. At this time, I was also advised to start having shallow salt baths to help heal the wounds on my buttocks and pubic area. It was so nice to be able to sit in a bath after only having showers for so long. I remember the first time I had a bath and being mesmerised by my new appendage bobbing around in the water. This made the whole unpleasant and painful surgery feel worthwhile! I wondered if natal born males were also fascinated with how their appendages bobbed around in the water, but I didn't care, I just owned it.

Chapter Fourteen - Spin Cycle

On the 22 January 2016, I saw Mr Christopher for the first time since leaving the hospital. He looked at my arm and phallus and remarked that I had an excellent result. He asked me if I had any sensation in my phallus and I told him that I was beginning to feel tactile sensation and was able to feel hot and cold water on it. He was very pleased and said that the nerves will take a long time to recover, but he was happy with the progress so far.

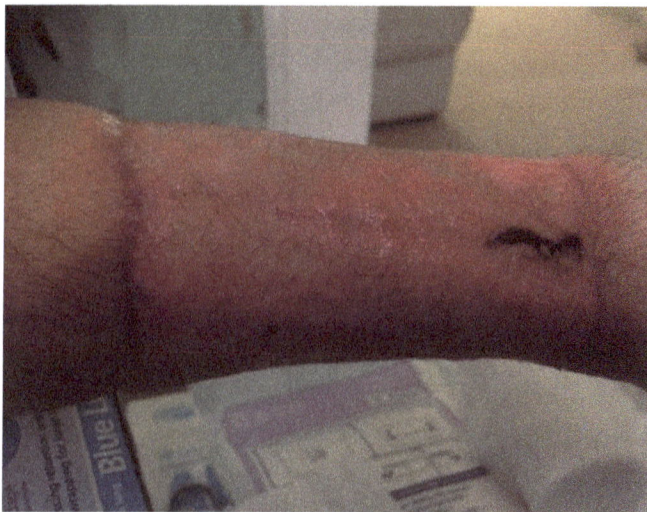

This is a picture of my arm, almost fully healed

At the end of the consultation, he said that I was ready for Stage Two which would be laparoscopic hysterectomy, join-up urethroplasty, burying of the clitoris, glans sculpting, vaginectomy and scrotoplasty. He said that because I was not working and was available at short-notice, they would try to give me the next date as soon as they could. I was thrilled that everything was going to plan and that there had been no major setbacks. I was mentally ready for Stage Two although, physically, I didn't feel as though my body had recovered; I felt as though I had just gone ten rounds with Mike Tyson. I was so glad that I didn't have to return to work too soon as I am not sure I would have coped. My job was very physical and, even with restricted duties, I would have struggled.

My relationship with Carla was going from strength to strength and she was a huge support to me along with both my Mum and Dad. Anyone going through gender confirmation surgery alone has to be applauded! I don't want to come across as patronising, but these surgeries are no walk in the park - they strip a person of everything, including their dignity. It's as if all of the organs are taken out of the body, put into a washing machine, put on the spin cycle and then put back into the person's body, while that person is still coping with all of the emotional stuff that goes with it.

A common misconception is that some people (a very small minority) think we bring this upon ourselves and therefore we should just get on with it. We do bring it upon ourselves, but we have little or no choice if we want to live a fulfilled and happy life in our correct gender. Also, just because we need these surgeries, it doesn't mean we are automatically equipped to cope with everything that they entail!

Because my relationship with Carla was going so well, we decided that we should move in together. Carla's ex was still living in their home near Heathrow and she refused to have me in the house. I wasn't surprised by this, as she saw me as the person that took Carla away from her. What she couldn't see was that she had been given every opportunity to fix their relationship, but she chose not to do this.

This was also Carla's home and she felt as if she had no say in the matter. I wouldn't have been comfortable going to the house when she was there anyway, so we decided that, for the sake of our relationship, we would move somewhere together where I could recover after surgery without the worry of her ex being around all the time.

We found a beautiful little flat in Tring, Hertfordshire, which was absolutely perfect. It was small, but it was all we needed for us and my soon-to-be adopted cat. We moved in and we made it our home and we were really happy there.

Whilst I was recovering, I did a bit of online shopping! I wanted to treat myself to a new car so that I had something to look forward to after surgery, even though I wouldn't be able to drive it immediately. After having looked around at some different showrooms online, I found myself a nice little sporty Audi- I was so excited!

Chapter Fifteen – Fire in the hole

I received my admission letter for Stage Two and, this time, I would be admitted to Spire Thames Valley Hospital on 9th July 2016. Stage Two, as previously mentioned, was vaginectomy, hysterectomy, join-up urethroplasty, burying of the clitoris, formation of the scrotum and glans sculpting. These procedures were to be carried out by another member of the London team and I would be in hospital for 2 days afterwards.

I was not looking forward to this stage because, although the surgery time was shorter and I wouldn't be in hospital for as long, I had been told that, post-op, the vaginectomy could be really painful. The reason for this is that light and heat are used to remove the tissue inside the vagina and the hole is then closed. I really didn't like the idea of the inside of my vagina being burned out, but it was what needed to be done.

A week before my procedure I visited the hospital for the same pre-op tests as had been done previously, with similar results. I was admitted to the hospital on the night before my procedure as per their requirement. I met the anaesthetist and the surgeon in the morning and nurses came in and out of my room preparing me for surgery. I was given the stockings to help prevent blood clots, the anti-bacterial wash and a gown. This time I was also given a tube of gel and I was asked to squirt some into each nostril; this is used as a precautionary measure as it has anti-bacterial properties.

I was told I would be second on the list and that they would tell me when I needed to start getting ready. For some reason, I was more nervous this time. I had got myself a little worked up because I had been told that I could be in quite a lot of pain afterwards. However, I was still excited to get Stage Two 'under my belt'.

As last time, we wandered around the ward for a while. The man in the next room to me was with someone who we presumed to be his girlfriend; they were chatting with the door open. Once again, Carla persuaded me to knock on the door and ask if we could come in for a chat. On entering the room, the first and most obvious thing seemed to be to ask if he was also having gender-confirming surgery. It was quite a difficult question to ask as, again, it is very intrusive and he may have been unwilling to share personal information with two strangers. He looked like a man, so we could have been completely wrong! There are a couple of things that are usually evident in most, but not all, Trans guys and that is the size of the hands and feet; Trans guys have smaller hands and feet because the original body was female.

Once we had got the awkwardness out of the way, we stayed chatting with them for quite some time and we got on really well. He seemed so chilled out and unconcerned about the surgery. He did tell me that he had decided not to have the vaginectomy part of the procedure, so perhaps that's why he wasn't too worried - either that, or he was very brave and I was a total wuss.

As he was going to theatre before me, we left him to get ready for his surgery and went back to my room. From that point forward, it felt as though time was standing still and that I was waiting for what seemed like forever. In reality, it really wasn't very long, as Stage Two normally only takes a few hours, not eight to ten like Stage One.

Eventually, the nurse came in and asked me to start getting prepared and told me that I would be going to theatre in about an hour. Once I had begun my preparations, the time seemed to vanish and, before I knew it, I was being taken to theatre.

Once again, the anaesthetist team was kind, and I think they could see how nervous I was. We shared some light banter whilst they inserted the cannula into my arm and gave me a pre-med. Once that had taken effect, I was given the anaesthetic and told to count down from ten. Again, I woke up bewildered in the recovery room and it felt as though I had only just been taken to surgery.

When I woke, I felt so sick, and because of my phobia about feeling or being sick, I asked one of the nurses for some anti-sickness medication. They told me that I had already had some in theatre, but that they would see if I could have some more. I was really feeling bad and was sure I was going to be sick. Fortunately, the nurse returned swiftly and said that I could have more medication and put it straight into the cannula- this helped quite quickly, and I was so relieved!

I spent the next hour or so in recovery because my blood-pressure and oxygen saturation were low. The nurse did an arterial blood-gas test which measures the amounts of arterial gases, such as oxygen and carbon dioxide. The blood is drawn from the radial artery and is tested to check that the body is moving oxygen around efficiently; this test also checks that carbon dioxide is being removed correctly. Imbalances in these levels can indicate certain medical conditions, but I think the team just wanted to ensure there was no underlying cause which was making my levels so low. All I remember is that this particular test was very painful even though I was still feeling light-headed from the anaesthetic!

Once these levels had begun to rise, I was taken to another room, but not my room. I was visited by one of the nurses who told me that I was in a room similar to an HDU (high dependency unit) and they wanted to keep me there until my blood-pressure and oxygen saturation had returned to a more normal level. By then I was so tired I didn't care where I was! A little while later, Carla and Mum came to see me; they had been so worried because they knew that the surgery only took a few hours, but I was gone for almost five! I was so pleased to see them as I was feeling a little sorry for myself.

Once all had returned to almost normal, I was taken back to my room, and the nurses checked on me hourly, to ensure that my levels had not dropped again. I still felt very sick but I was told I couldn't have any more anti-sickness medication as I had already been given the maximum dose.

I remember being in a lot of pain due to the vaginectomy part of the procedure. I could feel both burning and aching at the same time; it was horrible. The nurses were great and kept me topped up with pain relief as and when I needed it and, as had happened before, I also had a morphine® pump which I could control myself. The morphine® was good for pain relief, but I didn't use it very much as one of the side-effects is nausea or vomiting. I already felt so sick, and so I didn't want to make it worse.

I definitely felt much worse after this surgery than I did after the Stage One procedures. The vaginectomy and hysterectomy caused me a great deal of pain and, although, I was so grateful that it was over, it was not an easy recovery.

After a couple of days, it was time to be discharged, although I didn't feel at all ready. I was still in a considerable amount of pain and I wasn't sure how I was going to manage that at home. However, I did want to be at home where I could relax, and I was looking forward to returning to our little flat.

I had been sent home with a suprapubic catheter (a hollow tube that is inserted directly into the bladder just below the belly button), which is to allow urine to drain via a long tube, into a catheter bag. The catheter bag has to be placed lower to help the flow.

I was not yet able to urinate through my new urethra, because it still needed to heal. To assist with this, the catheter diverted the urine straight from the bladder, into the bag. I was also sent home with a urethral stent (a hollow tube that is inserted into the new urethra to keep it open and free from obstruction). I also had a dressing on my willy.

Both the stent and the dressing had to be removed by a district nurse, one-week post-surgery, so I made contact with the district nursing team to arrange for this to be done. Unfortunately, because I had moved from my parents' house, I was outside their catchment area. They did advise however, that if I could get myself to my own GP practice, one of the nurses could do this for me. However, I didn't know if I would be able to get to the doctors' surgery. Carla would have driven me there, but I would have needed to walk from the car park to the surgery, and that concerned me. I hoped that I would feel more able to do this nearer the appointment time. I made the appointment with one of the nurses at the surgery. I had already met her so she knew all about my transition, and I knew that I would feel comfortable with her doing what needed to be done.

Chapter Sixteen – Catheters: The Work of the Devil

The day came for my appointment with my GP, and Carla drove me to the surgery. Once there, we parked in a private car park that belonged to a local business. Obviously, the general public was not supposed to park there, but we had no choice as it was the nearest place to the surgery that we could find. A woman, who was also parking in the car park, wound down the window of her car and said "this is a private car park, you shouldn't be parking here". Carla told her that we had no choice as I had just had major surgery and there was nowhere close enough to park. Carla said that she would move the car once I was inside the GP practice. She wasn't impressed, but we walked off and left her to it. When Carla returned to move her car, the woman was still there and Carla told her, again, that I had just had very major surgery and that I was in pain and really couldn't walk very far. The woman then said that she was sorry she had been so unpleasant, but so many people parked there when they shouldn't.

Once in the nurse's room, I sat down and told her all about my surgery. She was so interested and couldn't wait to see the results! She asked me to undress and to lie on the couch so that she could take off the dressing and remove the stent. She was absolutely 'gobsmacked' when she saw my new appendage and said that it was an amazing result. She also said "that's a good size!" That probably would have been inappropriate in any 'normal' situation, but because we had a good relationship, it was totally acceptable to me. It was also a nice confidence booster.

She removed the dressing on the glans and said that it was healing very well and, as per the post-op instruction sheet that she had received, she redressed this with Mepitel. Removal of the stent requires deflating a balloon, which is the method used for holding the tube in the correct place and ensuring that it doesn't come out. Although it wasn't too painful, it felt weird, as though a worm was wiggling under the skin. I was pleased to have the stent removed, as it was a little annoying having this tube hanging out of my willy. The supra-pubic catheter was to remain in place for a further two weeks.

Carla's daughter came to Tring to visit us for a few days. One night, I had a problem with my supra-pubic catheter which had become blocked. It had stopped flowing on one other occasion, but I was able to re-position it to re-start the flow. But this time I was unable to get it flowing again and I could feel my bladder becoming full, which was extremely uncomfortable. I began to panic and I decided that I would cut the tube to allow the urine to flow out. I had no idea of what I was doing and I managed to cut the tube in the wrong place! This meant that the urine didn't start flowing again and also that the catheter was now useless. I called Mr Christopher and explained the situation. I was so embarrassed about what I had done, but he said I was definitely not the first person to have done it and I wouldn't be the last. I asked for his advice and he told me to get myself to A&E as I could end up with a blocked bladder, a condition that is not only dangerous, but extremely uncomfortable. He told me that they would need to empty my bladder, flush it and then re-catheterise.

We arrived at A&E and I was told to sit in the waiting area. I was panicking because my bladder was filling up and it was so uncomfortable. We waited for about half an hour at which point Carla went back to the reception desk and asked how much longer I would be waiting. She told the receptionist that I had just had major surgery and that I needed to be seen quickly. The receptionist told her that they were very busy and that I would be seen as soon as possible. We waited a further twenty minutes, by which point, it felt like my bladder was so full, it was going to burst. Once again, Carla went back to the receptionist and said that they needed to see me now! She was told to go through to the treatment area and speak to one of the doctors. When she returned, she told me that the doctor had said to bring me through to him.

Once in the treatment area, we were told to go into one of the bays and I was asked to remove my clothes. Carla's daughter had come with us and, if I hadn't been in so much discomfort, I would have been extremely embarrassed, as I was lying naked on the bed! She was great, though and she didn't make me feel awkward.

I waited in there for what seemed like another lifetime. When the doctor arrived, she asked me for some medical history relating to the surgery I had undergone. She then asked me what I wanted her to do about this situation. We all looked at each other in disbelief and then I turned to the doctor and said "I think my bladder needs to be emptied and flushed, and then you will need to re-catheterise me!" The doctor said that she didn't really know the protocol for this situation given that I was a Trans patient.

I had already known that there was little (or no) training given to medical professionals on gender-confirming surgeries. I tried to be patient with the doctor, but ended up getting frustrated because I was suffering. I said "surely, it would be the same protocol if a man came into hospital with a catheter that had blocked". The doctor was a little bemused by my comment and said that she would have to contact my surgeon so that she could be talked through the procedure. It was around 10pm and I couldn't believe that she was suggesting that she needed to speak to Mr Christopher before doing anything. I didn't even know if he would answer his phone at this time of night. Thankfully, he did!

I could hear most of what Mr Christopher was saying to the doctor and he sounded a little shocked to hear that this couldn't be dealt with without consulting him. Regardless of this, with great patience he talked her through what needed to be done.

The doctor managed to draw out the urine via a syringe and emptied my bladder. She then flushed it to clean it all out and finally re-catheterised me. The re-catheterisation was painful but what a relief it was to have an empty bladder! Emptying one's bladder is probably something that we all take for granted as a normal function, so to not be able to do this was horrible. I couldn't wait to have this catheter finally removed as it was causing me so many problems.

I continued to regain strength and mobility but, unfortunately, late one night, the catheter again became blocked. I didn't want a repeat of what happened the last time in A&E, so I called the hospital where I had the surgery. I spoke to a nurse on the ward and asked her if I could come in to have the catheter flushed. She wasn't overly keen on the idea, as normally they wouldn't deal with these post-operative issues. She did finally agree to let me come in to save me having to go to A&E. She advised me to come to the hospital and ring on the doorbell as the ward would be closed.

On arrival, I was shown into a side room and seen fairly quickly by one of the nurses. He knew exactly what to do which made things so much easier for me. He quickly flushed the catheter and made sure it was running again before sending me on my way.

In the week leading up to the removal of the supra-pubic catheter, I had been advised to get a flip-flow valve which inserts into the end of the tube that would normally go into the catheter bag. The reason for using the flip-flow valve is to allow retraining of the bladder, after having had a catheter for a period of time. When a catheter is attached to a bag, the bladder doesn't ever become full as it is constantly draining. This means that the bladder needs to be 'retrained' to allow you to know when it is full, so that it can then be emptied. To operate the valve, it must be turned to the open position to evacuate the urine; when the bladder is empty, the valve must be closed. Unfortunately, as the catheter sits against the bladder wall, when there is no more urine present, the bladder will spasm - this is not pleasant! Fortunately, this procedure is only in use for the last week before the catheter is removed entirely.

There was a week or so left before I could have the catheter removed, but I was desperate to get this thing out. I called St. Peters Andrology centre and asked one of the nurses if I could have the catheter removed early. She said that it needed to remain in-situ for the full period of time recommended by the surgeon. I told her about all the problems that I had been experiencing, but she wouldn't change her mind. I was determined to get the catheter removed one way or another, so I called Mr Christopher and asked him to consider my request; he took a lot of persuading, but he finally agreed.

I booked an appointment at St. Peters Andrology Clinic to see one of the nurses for the catheter removal. On the day of my appointment, I saw a nurse that I had met before and I told her all about the problems I was having. She told me that it was common with this type of catheter and she didn't blame me for wanting it gone. I was asked to lie on the couch and to take a deep breath in whist she deflated the balloon and pulled out the catheter. This was definitely more uncomfortable than having the stent removed but, finally, IT WAS OUT! She gave me an antibiotic injection to prevent infection and told me to sit in the waiting area and drink plenty of water as, before I could leave the clinic, I had to make sure that I could void (urinate through my phallus).

This was the first time I would be doing this so I was nervous, but excited. I had no idea of what to expect, how it would feel or if I would get my aim right. It was going to be a profound experience and one that I had wanted for so long but I didn't feel prepared. With all that said, it went very well and I even managed to get most of the pee in the toilet. It was such a strange sensation to feel the urine going down the tube (urethra), but to see it coming out of the end of my willy was the icing on the cake. For the first time in my life, I felt whole.

Unfortunately, this was not the end of my troubles post Stage Two. I was recovering well and had finally begun to feel more human apart from the fact that I felt so sick all of the time. I actually think I don't cope very well with anaesthesia but, apart from that, everything else was going well. Until one day, I woke up in incredible pain. I couldn't pinpoint exactly where the pain was coming from, but it seemed to be coming from the vaginectomy site; the pain was so bad, I was crying. Carla didn't know what to do for me as I had already tried pain medication, but it had no effect.

Unfortunately, it was a weekend and the Andrology Clinic was closed, so Carla called 111. The operator said that they wouldn't send an ambulance because Carla could drive me to A&E. Even after Carla asked how I was supposed to walk down the stairs from the flat, they still said we would have to make our own way. I was in so much pain, but we were given no choice, we just had to make our own way there.

I managed to get to the car with a lot of help from Carla and then spent the entire journey in agony. When we got to A&E, we were asked to wait again, for what seemed like all of eternity. Finally, we were called in to see a doctor. The doctor asked me for a brief history and also for the reason I had come to A&E. I explained about my recent surgery and told him that I had never experienced pain like this. Yet again, I was asked "what would you like me to do about this?" Carla and I looked at each other with disbelief and then Carla said "you are the doctor, why are you asking us?" He looked puzzled, and almost shocked, by her response.

Carla explained that we had experienced issues with a lack of knowledge around the protocols for dealing with Trans patients experiencing post-operative problems. She said that it wasn't acceptable that someone who is going through gender confirming surgery who presents with a medical problem, like severe pain, would not be treated in the same way as anyone else. She was pretty angry, but she did say that this was down to a lack of training and not his fault.

The doctor said that the most he could do was to prescribe me some morphine® and that I should go and get myself checked by my surgeon. Given that he was a healthcare professional, neither of us liked his demeanour; he was unsympathetic and had no clue how to talk to people. I left the hospital with a small bottle of Oramorph® and we went home. After another extremely painful journey, we arrived at our flat. I had already taken a dose of the Oramorph which normally works quickly due to the fact that it is in liquid form rather than tablet form, but it didn't even take the edge off the pain.

It suddenly occurred to me to put a post on the surgery group that I had joined, to ask for some advice. Within a few minutes someone replied saying that if we emailed St. Peters Andrology Clinic, the email would be redirected to a surgeon and, because it was an emergency, a surgeon would make contact.

We were both so relieved to hear this and I quickly sent an email. Within about ten minutes, Mr Christopher had called me and said that I would need to go to the Spire Thames Valley hospital so that he could see me. Luckily for me; he was actually working in the hospital on that day. He told me not to eat anything in case I needed to have surgery.

I was in so much pain, I didn't care that we had to go back out again, I just wanted some relief. When we arrived at the hospital, I was taken to a room so that I would be more comfortable. Mr Christopher came to see me shortly after this. I explained the pain and from where it seemed to originate, and he told me it was most likely to be a vaginal abscess which would need to be drained. He would need to do a Cystoscopy (insertion of a flexible tube with a camera on the end) and then drain the vaginal abscess cavity and, unfortunately, this would have to be done under anaesthetic.

I really didn't want to undergo another anaesthetic, but I was relieved to hear that something could be done to get rid of the pain. I was prepared for surgery and within about an hour was in theatre.

I came around after the surgery and, although I was still groggy from the anaesthetic, the first thing I noticed was that the pain had gone - what a relief! Mr Christopher came to visit me that evening before he left the hospital and he told me that I did have an abscess and that it was successfully drained. He said that it had been necessary to re-catheterise me, both with a supra-pubic catheter and a urethral catheter. I was really unhappy that I had the supra-pubic catheter in again as this is the one that caused me so many issues last time. I also had a Yates drain placed into my vagina. This is a drain used when there is a need for sustained and constant drainage, and it was needed to ensure that any pus would be able to drain from the cavity.

Carla asked him what would have happened if he hadn't come in and he said that the abscess could have burst which could potentially lead to blood poisoning (sepsis).I felt extremely fortunate that I had avoided this potential outcome, but things could have been very different if I had not posted on the surgery group.

I left the hospital the next day and was given a discharge letter that outlined the post-operative care I would need. The drain would need to be removed in one week and the urethral catheter would need to stay in place for three weeks unless it became intolerable, and then it could be removed after ten days. The supra-pubic catheter would also need to stay in for three weeks, by which time everything should have settled and healed and I could go back to the clinic to have a trial void.

Fortunately, I didn't have the same issues with the supra-pubic catheter this time, other than the fact that it was horribly uncomfortable. Once again, I managed to negotiate with Mr Christopher to have the catheters removed a little earlier than he had recommended.

With no catheters in place, I was able, once again, to urinate through my willy, and I was feeling so much better. I had been 'through the mill' with Stage Two and I was glad that things were finally settling, so that I could prepare myself for Stage Three.

Chapter Seventeen - New Equipment

In September 2016, I had a phone conversation with the clinic, to discuss my recovery and my suitability to be added to the surgical waiting list for Stage Three. Mr Christopher had already said that I would probably be ready for this, sometime around February 2017. The nurse told me that, provided that everything was still ok when we had our next telephone call, I would be added to the list.

I continued to recover well and loved the fact that I was able to pee standing up which, to me, was the epitome of masculinity. I would often go to the toilet even if I didn't need to go because I wanted to use my new equipment. I never thought peeing could be so much fun!

The nurse from the clinic called to say that she was happy with my progress and that I would now be put on the list for my final surgery. Although this made me feel very happy, I was also anxious because of all I had been through. However, I knew that this was the last piece of the puzzle, so over the next few months I tried to prepare myself mentally for the final hurdle.

Carla and I were still living in our little flat in Tring and our relationship was growing stronger and stronger. She was my rock, standing beside me through everything and for that I will be eternally grateful. Again, my thoughts were with anyone who goes through all of this without support from someone close; I couldn't imagine having gone through all of my experiences without Carla. Not only are there physical care needs, there are also emotional ones. Carla told me that she found it very difficult to cope at times, even though she was not the one going through it all. She said that seeing someone she loves going so much pain was horrible!

Before I knew it, the awaited letter from the nurse at the clinic arrived, advising me that my final surgery would take place on 20th March 2017 at St. John and St. Elizabeth hospital. This surgery was for the insertion of an inflatable penile prosthesis. Mr Christopher had already told me which device he would probably use (Coloplast Titan® with QS8n pump) and that he would only use one inflatable tube inside, due to the space inside my phallus not being large enough for two.

By the time I received this letter, I felt ready to take on the final stage, as I knew that very soon it would all be over and I would be able to get on with enjoying the rest of my life.

As on previous occasions, I was admitted to hospital the night before the procedure and I was settled into my room. I recognised some of the nurses from previous admissions, and it was comforting to see familiar faces.

On the following morning, all of the normal preparations for surgery took place, and Mr Christopher came to see me. He told me that, after the penile prosthesis was inserted, he would inflate it using the pump. The reason for this is to ensure that it is working correctly and also to give the phallus time to adjust to having something inflated inside the space. He advised that it would need to remain inflated (erect) for at least one-week post op. This caused a few giggles as I imagined having to walk around with an erection.

I was told that I would be third on the list and, although this meant I would be waiting for a while, that was okay. I had Carla, my rock, with me and she helped me to pass the time. When the time arrived for my surgery, I remember thinking - this is it, the final stage. The next thing I remembered was waking up in the recovery room and just smiling to myself- it was over! As with the previous surgeries, my blood-pressure was rather low, but this time it didn't seem to cause too much concern and I was taken back to my room fairly quickly. This procedure was the shortest surgery of all the three stages and was the least invasive, so I was due to be discharged the following day. The next morning, I was given some post op instructions and sent on my way.

I remember thinking, how the hell am I going to leave the hospital with, for want of a better word, a 'boner'. Once we had packed my bags, we left the ward with me clutching a bag in front of my groin area. Although I had on the baggiest pair of jogging bottoms I could find, I was still conscious that people would see the protrusion. Finally, we made it out of the hospital without managing to attract any strange looks!

I spent the following week resting and recovering but I really didn't want to go out as it would have been too embarrassing. I was looking forward to having the prosthesis deflated so that I could leave the flat and not worry that my appendage might be the centre of attention.

I had been warned that the first deflation can sometimes be extremely painful and I was advised to take some pain-killers before my appointment so, on the morning of the appointment, I took some codeine and paracetamol and hoped that it would help me.

Carla took me to the clinic and I was met by the same nurse that I had seen previously. She asked if I had taken any pain-killers; she said that, in her experience and according to feedback, the deflation can be extremely painful. She said that some people tolerate it better than others, but that it also depended on the amount of swelling in the testicle around the pump. I told her that I had taken pain relief, as advised, because I have low pain tolerance.

The nurse asked me to lie on the bed and said that Carla could sit with me for moral support. She checked the wounds first and said that everything was healing well and that the cylinder inside my phallus was in a good position, with no signs of erosion. There are two controls on the pump, one to inflate the cylinder and one to deflate it. When she tried to locate the deflation device, she had some difficulty because it had moved. It is quite common for this to happen as the pump settles in after surgery. She said that there was still some swelling around the pump and told me that it was probably going to be quite painful. Oh boy, I was not looking forward to this at all! It was painful enough already with just her trying to locate the deflation device.

Carla took my hand so that I could squeeze it if I needed to. Once the nurse had managed to get the deflation device between her fingers, she told me to take a deep breath so that she could deflate it. Well, I nearly hit the roof, the pain was excruciating! Carla told me that her hand had turned white because I was squeezing it so hard! I tried so hard to relax because I knew that it needed to be done. The nurse tried twice more, but said that it was difficult because the device moves around and makes it hard to get it into the right place.

I couldn't cope with her trying anymore and told her that I might have to come back on another day. She agreed that the swelling was making it too painful and said that she would make an appointment a week later to try again when the swelling should have reduced.

Another week passed and I was back on the bed in the nurses' room; I really wasn't looking forward to this at all. Luckily for me, this time she located the pump quickly and, although it was still really painful, she managed to deflate it- what a relief! She told me that my next appointment would be in about three weeks and that would be to show me how to inflate and deflate the pump myself- this is called cycling.

When the time came for my appointment, I was feeling so much better and I knew that the swelling around the pump and testicle had reduced, as it was not so uncomfortable. I was looking forward to what would, hopefully, be my last trip to the clinic. Finally, I would be able to see and feel what it was like to experience an erection, albeit with the aid of a pump.

The appointment went without a hitch and the nurse was able to show me how to locate the two areas on the pump and to instruct me on how to use it. Even though the swelling had reduced, I was only able to cycle the pump once as it was still quite painful.

Whilst there, I asked for some advice as I was experiencing some itching around the base of the scrotum. She explained that this might be due to the pooling of urine in the new urethra. This can happen because urine is acidic and if the urethra isn't fully drained, skin irritation can be the result. She showed me a technique called 'milking', which is as it sounds. The technique is used to squeeze out any urine that may be sitting in the bend of the urethra. She said that this would probably help with the irritation and that it would also help to prevent leaking, post-urination.

When the appointment was over, I experienced a moment of pure clarity- this was everything that I had been waiting for. I had fully transitioned from female to male and now I felt male in every sense. This had been the toughest journey I had ever been on but, finally, I was whole.

Chapter Eighteen - Yes Ma'am, No Ma'am

Over the course of the next few months, Carla and I remained in our little flat in Tring. I was still recovering, but I really needed some mental stimulation. I had often thought about training to become a counsellor, but I had not yet committed to doing it. There were many reasons for this, but the one that stands out is my lack of confidence. Carla had always told me that she thought I should do the training as I have natural empathy and some good life experiences, but I had always found excuses not to do it. Now that I had time on my hands and I was feeling much more confident, I decided to begin the process of training to become a counsellor.

I applied to the college where Carla had done her training, as she recommended it and said that the tutors were excellent. Once enrolled, I felt a sense of achievement, as I felt that I would be doing something positive which could change my life and the lives of others.

The courses were difficult, requiring a lot of coursework but I managed to complete the first two stages in the process. I know that I work in a structured and methodical way, and I do very well in written assignments or essays. However, I knew that I would find the last part of the process the hardest, as it involved a large amount of evidence-based coursework and, also, a lot of practice counselling sessions.

The coursework would have been hard and, probably, I would have been comfortable with that, but the practical sessions worried me. I had done some of these sessions in the first two courses and they always scared the crap out of me! I would get so worked up beforehand even though I actually did well in the sessions and I knew that, if I wanted to be a counsellor, I would have to get over this and 'feel the fear and do it anyway'

I also knew that I needed some help to try to work out why I was so anxious about these sessions, so I began seeing a private talking therapy counsellor. I had a few appointments with her, and we tried to get to the route of my problem.

During these sessions, I came to my own conclusion; my fears were based around failure. I don't know why I had these fears because I had never failed at anything. Whatever I decided to undertake, I achieved with great results. We talked about what failure meant to me when thinking of becoming a qualified counsellor and I told her that I just didn't think I would be good enough. We never really got to the bottom of this, but she did have a positive impact on my general wellbeing.

As I was nearing the end of the second course, I was already beginning to talk myself out of doing the last part. Both my tutor and my colleagues were full of praise and encouragement, but I couldn't seem to get over this fear. I think a lot of my previous confidence issues were fear-related and this situation was no different. Although I had gained so much confidence through the transition process, I still had doubts about myself that even the counsellor couldn't help to dispel. Unfortunately, I didn't go on to qualify as a counsellor; I just couldn't bring myself to do it.

After having lived in the flat for around six months, we came to the realisation that it was not fair for Carla to continue to pay her contribution to the mortgage on her house. Her ex was still living there and we were also paying rent on the flat. We decided that Carla would contact her ex to tell her that both she and I would be moving to the house and that it was up to her if she wanted to stay there. Her ex told her that there was absolutely no way that she would remain in the house with both of us living there and she would be moving out; this was exactly what we wanted her to say. We gave our notice on the flat and made plans to move back to Heathrow.

After our notice period, we moved to the house which is where we remained until December 2019. Carla was so pleased to be back in her home again and we made some superficial changes to the décor which made it feel more homely for both of us, however it never really felt like my home.

Carla and I went through another little bump in the road after having been back at the house for a while. As I have already mentioned, Carla had always identified as a Lesbian - she had just chosen to be in a relationship with me, which slotted her nicely into society's tick-box of being in a heterosexual relationship. However, she was clearly struggling with certain aspects of the way I looked - I was male after all and she liked the female form.

It was during an evening out with some friends, that this became evident, even without any words being spoken about it. We all had had a fair bit to drink that evening and I could see that Carla was getting rather close to one of our friends. The evening was coming to an end and I saw Carla going in to the toilet after this friend and I was pretty sure that they would probably kiss. I never did question her about it as although I knew it in my head, I almost didn't want confirmation of it.

The next day Carla told me that we needed to talk about what had happened and how she was feeling. The talk resulted in Carla asking me for some space and time to allow her to process how she was feeling.

This was so difficult for me because I thought we were so good together and it worried me that, once again, I might find myself on my own again. It was a huge blow to my confidence and almost cemented the thoughts I had had earlier in my transition- 'who is going to want to be with me?'

I gave Carla the space she needed, although this was really hard for me and I am glad I did. Over time she realised that what was important to her was the love she had for me as a person and that she would rather have that.

We both wanted to begin our new life together in a home which we would buy together, one which hadn't been lived in with any ex-partners. I had always envisaged living in the country and I wanted us to make a home together, somewhere away from London. I grew up in London and although I had experienced some happy times there,

I wanted to move to somewhere more tranquil. It was food for thought and something we talked about quite regularly.

As we continued our journey together, I was settling into life as a man and adapting to ever-changing scenarios. Although I had lived for two years as a male before starting my surgical transition, I was still very much learning what it was to be a man.

I was no longer being mis-gendered; the only time this did happen was on the telephone. My voice had dropped significantly after being on T for a few years but, clearly, it hadn't dropped enough. I would often have to correct people on the telephone when they called me Miss or Ma'am. I would be asked if I was the account holder as they would see the name on my account as Daniel, but to them I sounded female. This was really embarrassing and frustrating- had I really been through this nightmare of a journey to be put through this? I had to learn to accept that this might be the way it could be for the rest of my life!

I learned that, even though I was male, I felt more comfortable in the company of women. This had also been the case pre-transition and there is nothing wrong with that, but I actually felt, and still feel, awkward around other men.

I also began to experience something that a good friend of mine had told me about- male privilege. Apparently, this describes the way men are treated by other men. A man will tend to address another man first, even if he has a woman by his side. I am not entirely sure why this happens and I don't actually like the notion at all. Unfortunately, it is just one of those things that seem to happen naturally.

One thing that I will never get used to is the horror of men's public toilets; they smell disgusting and are generally very unpleasant! I much preferred using ladies' toilets, which meant not having to worry about what I am wading through to get to the toilet. However, using men's urinals gives me a buzz, as does having the ability to pee outside (in the countryside, of course); no more worrying about peeing down my legs or on my shoes and there are no more concerns about being stung by stinging nettles in the nether regions!

I loved the way that I was being accepted as a man, especially by other men. Being called Mr or Sir to my face, was so affirming that it made everything feel right and as if it had always been that way. Even though I knew myself to be male, to be seen in this way by others was amazing!

A by-product of my transition is that it has given me so much more confidence. I was, and probably always will be, a little shy when I meet new people, but because I am so much more comfortable with myself and my body, I have become more confident. I began to think about doing things that I would never have considered pre-transition.

I knew that I wanted to give something back to society and, in particular, to the Trans community, so Carla and I put together a workshop which we could use to help people understand what it means to be Transgender. One of the main things which we had learned during my transition experience, was that there was a lack of training and understanding of what Trans people go through to feel fulfilled in every aspect of their lives. We designed a training talk which could easily be adapted for any group.

The sessions involved talking through a number of slides, giving factual information and interactive learning. I created a video showing images of my transition and, alongside this, I told my own story. We decided that we wouldn't charge anything for our time in providing these workshops as this was our way of 'paying it forward', using our knowledge and our experiences to help others.

One of the areas that we concentrated on was counselling and counsellors. Carla is a trained therapeutic counsellor and, previously, I had also completed a Certificate and a Level 2 in Counselling Skills, so we knew this would be a great place to start.

Counsellors see a wide range of people with varying problems and if they were to come across anyone who was Trans, the workshop would give them a base of knowledge; although they would already have natural empathy, they would also have an understanding or a real sense of what someone experiences during transition.

Carla's former tutor invited us to her NVQ Level Three counselling classes so that we could run our workshop. The training was really well received and the students were so grateful for the experience. The feedback that we received was fantastic and everyone said that, prior to attending this session, they really had no idea what was involved in transition. The tutor was so impressed that she asked us back to do the same workshop for another group of her students.

My Mum is a Samaritan and she also asked us to run a workshop for her branch. As with counsellors, there is a possibility that Samaritan volunteers may come across a caller who is Trans. We ran our workshop for them and, once again, the feedback was fantastic. We spoke to some of the attendees afterward and they told us that they felt they had acquired some real insight into the life of someone who is Trans, and that it had helped them to understand some of the potential issues that someone may have to deal with.

Chapter Nineteen - Wedding Bells

I had reached the stage where I felt comfortable in my new skin and I was ready to return to the world of work. I managed to find a job at a hotel that was a ten-minute drive from home. The job was something completely new to me as I had never before worked in hospitality but, because part of the job was office-based, I felt slightly out of my comfort zone. I had never worked in an office but I was looking forward to a new challenge. I might not have considered doing this work pre-transition, as I didn't think I had the required confidence to do the job well, but as part of this job was to assist in the running of the conference department, I felt that this would help to further build that confidence. The job was everything I hoped it would be and I met some wonderful people there who soon became friends. I didn't tell everyone there about my transition, but I told the people with whom I felt comfortable and I couldn't have hoped for a more supportive reaction.

Carla and I had been discussing getting married as, although we were engaged, we had yet to set a wedding date. We finally decided to have a small civil ceremony on the 24th September 2019 as neither of us was religious. We wanted this to take place at our local Registry Office with only close family in attendance. We planned to have another ceremony on 25th October 2019, which was to be a Humanist wedding service, and this was going to be the main event as we would have all our family and friends with us.

I had decided on the person I wanted to have as my best man and Carla was happy with my decision. I wanted this to be the friend I had met at the support group, as he and his family had become an integral part of mine and Carla's lives, and I wouldn't have wanted anyone else to be my best man. He said that he would be honoured to support me, and that it had made him so happy to be asked. I was thrilled that he had accepted and I couldn't wait to have him by my side on our wedding day.

We both decided that we wanted our little dog Charlie to be our ring bearer. We were so excited by the thought of our little furry one running down the aisle with our rings attached to her collar.

The planning for our wedding came at a particularly busy time as we were also organising a home move, and dealing with both events at the same time made it very stressful for us both. Not only was all this happening, but I had also just discovered that, in order to be married as a man and not a woman, I would need to apply to the Gender Recognition Panel for a Gender Recognition Certificate (GRC). We didn't have much time to organise this, so I had to come to terms with the fact that I may have had to, legally, marry as a woman.

The application process for this certificate can take a long time and a great deal of information must be submitted to the GR Processing Team for review. Only when all of the required documentation is received by them will a date be set for a hearing with the Gender Recognition Panel, which decides whether the individual applying is to be known by their chosen gender. I found this process frustrating and slightly humiliating! Who are these people to decide whether someone they have never met, is male or female? Unfortunately, this was the process and I had to adhere to it.

I was very relieved when I received confirmation that they had all the required paperwork to set a hearing date, as this meant that there was a chance that I might have the certificate before the legal marriage was due to take place. However, the hearing date was very close to the date of the wedding, which meant that there might not be enough time to get the marriage documents amended. I really wanted things to go as smoothly as possible, so I called the Processing Team and asked them about the likelihood of receiving the certificate before the wedding date. They were very honest with me and said that it would depend on how quickly the paperwork was sent out after the hearing and this would be on the assumption that the panel would grant the certificate. The woman I spoke to was so helpful and said that she would do whatever she could to expedite the process for me. Patience has never been my strongest attribute, but I had no choice but to wait and hope that I would be issued with a GRC and that it would arrive before the big day.

During, and after, my transition I had gained some weight which I carried mainly around my hips and buttocks. I didn't like the way this made me look, or feel, because I had a very different image of what masculinity was and I thought I didn't fit this image. I made a decision to seek help from a professional PT (physical trainer).

One day, whilst having my haircut, I was chatting to my barber and he mentioned that his brother-in-law was an online PT with his own company called V2 Fitness (Version 2 fitness). His name was Salvatore Bruno but most people called him Bruno. He told me to look at his website and see what I thought and, if I was happy to go ahead, he would refer me so that I could get a discount.

A few weeks later, I took the plunge and contacted Bruno to see what he could offer me. We had a long chat about my primary goals and what I wanted to achieve. My first goal was to lose weight for my wedding. He said that this would be a great first goal and that it would be completely achievable by that date.

I told him all about my transition so that he would be able to adapt a programme to suit my needs. He was extremely helpful; he told me that there would be no difference in how he would train me as compared with how he would train someone that hadn't transitioned, as the principles were the same.

I had always hated going to gyms. I found it boring and full of people who looked amazing, but I was now looking forward to the challenge of creating a more masculine body. Bruno had made me feel completely at ease on the phone and he was full of praise and admiration for the journey I had taken. From the outset, he was so enthusiastic and that filled me with confidence. I came off the phone with such a positive mind-set and a new found energy for the next part of my journey.

Over the next few months, I trained hard and I also followed Bruno's advice about nutrition; I was starting to see some desperately needed results. One thing I know about myself, it is that I perform really well when I have targets to meet, be that in a work situation or in my personal life. I am at my best when I have focus, structure and routine, and these are all of the things that Bruno helped me to practice.

Even though it was tough, I was able to maintain my workout routine alongside my full-time job. I kept a log of my daily calorie intake and uploaded all my workout sessions onto an app. The app was a great tool to help me to stay focussed on my goals. I also had weekly telephone check-ins with Bruno, during which we would discuss my week.

These weekly calls were essential to me as, without that accountability, I would have struggled. I knew that if I 'fell off the wagon' I would be letting myself down and I felt that I would also be letting Bruno down. In fact, I couldn't have been more wrong; if there were setbacks or struggles or situations that meant that I couldn't work out, Bruno would never focus on them. He would tell me that tomorrow would be a new day and I should move on. If I had demolished a whole pizza or eaten my own body weight in pasta, there would be no scolding, he would just encourage me to try again. Bruno made the difference between me winning or losing and I was most definitely winning. I had managed to lose 11kg before my wedding day, and I looked and felt great.

On the 24th September, Carla and I were married at the Registry Office and, luckily for me, I had received the GRC on the day before the legal marriage was to take place. The Registrar had already said it might be too late to change the paperwork, so I might have to be married as a woman.

Carla managed to get the GRC to the Registrar the day before the ceremony and she said that she would do her very best to have the paperwork amended for the next day.

Later that day, Carla received a call from the Registrar saying that she had been able to amend the paperwork and that I would be, legally, marrying as a man. When Carla finished talking to the Registrar, she was very excited as she told me the good news and, of course, I was thrilled.

On the day of the ceremony, we met the Registrar and she was very pleased that she would be marrying me as a man. We thanked her profusely, as without her determination to help us, it would have been a different story.

The ceremony was lovely considering it was just the legal part of our marriage and the Registrar did such a great job. We were both now looking forward to the Humanist Ceremony where we could celebrate with all our family and friends.

Over the next month, we concentrated on finalising all the details in preparation for the big event and when the time came for us to be married again, we were both really excited; this was it, the day we had been planning for so long. When I say we had been planning, most of the wedding was actually planned by Carla and her daughter Lou. I played my part but, without them, I would have been lost.

We spent the night apart as Carla wanted to keep the long-standing tradition where the bride doesn't see the groom until she walks down the aisle. I thought I would be more nervous on the day but, I think, because we had already been legally married, I felt as though I had been given a practice run.

The time had come! Our family and friends gathered before taking their seats for the ceremony and I had my 'main man' by my side; I was so proud of him.

The Humanist Celebrant who married us was amazing and the ceremony was fantastic and also emotional, and was just what we both had wanted.

Charlie played her part amazingly well and bounded down the aisle to deliver our rings. She was so excited and got a great welcome from our guests.

We spent the evening in the company of our truly amazing family and friends and couldn't have had a better day. It was perfect in every way.

Chapter Twenty - Onward and Upward

I stayed at my new job for almost a year and a half before Carla and I finally took the plunge and made the decision to move out of London to the country. We had already spoken to my parents about moving away and, although they were completely supportive, they would have preferred us to remain closer to them; they said that it was for selfish reasons that they really wanted us to live nearer to them, which we completely understood. Ideally, we would have loved to live near them in Hertfordshire but, unfortunately, property in that area was too expensive for us.

As Carla's ex had retained part ownership of the house near Heathrow, we had to ensure that the amount we would receive from its sale would be enough to allow us, not only to buy her out but also, to enable us to move on ourselves.

We spent a great deal of time deciding on the area where we wanted to live, trying to keep the distance between us and my parents as short as possible. We quickly discovered that the further away from London we looked, the cheaper property prices became and this had to be a consideration, as we hoped to be mortgage free, or to have as small a mortgage as was possible. We viewed places in Somerset, Devon and Wiltshire and eventually found a lovely bungalow in Somerset in a not too rural location, close enough to areas of natural beauty to be able to walk there.

We also chose this area as, within a twenty-five-minute drive, we could be in Devon and Dorset so, not only would we live in a beautiful country location, we would also be able to access the Jurassic coast and other coastal destinations.

Carla tried to negotiate with her ex, the proportion of equity she would receive when the house was sold. Carla had lived in that house for many years before her ex moved in with her and so we both felt that she should not be entitled to half of the equity. After taking legal advice, we decided that we wouldn't insist on this course of action as it might have meant going to court, and neither of us wanted this, we just wanted to move on.

We were able to secure a small mortgage which would allow us to purchase a property in Somerset and still have money left over to do any works that were needed. Once we had secured the mortgage, we began to plan our move.

I handed in my notice at my job, but we decided that Carla would remain at her job as her work could be flexible and would allow her to work from home. We moved to Somerset in December 2019 and it was the best decision we could have made; it is such a beautiful place.

After the move, I took a few months before I started to look for work so that I could do some things at the new property. Once the works had been completed, I started to look for a job and managed to find one working as a receptionist at a solicitors' practice in Taunton. My initial job interview went very well and I received a call a few days later asking me to go into the office to meet one of the other partners, before they made their final decision. I got on really well with my interviewers and I knew that I was going to fit in. I was offered the job immediately after my second interview.

Over the next few weeks, I settled into my new job; I really liked the people there and I enjoyed my role. Unfortunately, I had only been working there for about a month when, on March 23rd 2020, the country went into lock-down due to Covid-19, the deadly pandemic that began at the end of 2019

I was asked to go into furlough, a Government scheme set up to assist companies to retain their employees and enable them to be paid 80% of their salaries, until the crisis was over. Unfortunately, as I had been with the company for only a short time, I didn't qualify for this scheme. Like many others, I was left wondering how I would pay the household bills.

One of the practice partners regularly kept me updated on the situation and he said that the practice would fight my case to try to get me included in the scheme. After a week, I received a call from him saying that the rules set out by the Government were very strict and, as I hadn't been on the company payroll by the designated date, I was not eligible; this was really worrying!

He asked me how this outcome would affect me financially. I was very honest with him and I said that, although it wouldn't put us on the breadline, as Carla was still working from home, I knew that it would be a real struggle.

I told him that we had recently moved and had completed some house renovations, and we still had our mortgage and other bills to pay. He told me that the company would not leave me without any payment and that they would do all that they could to help me.

I knew that Covid-19 would have a huge impact on many businesses, so I thought that they were being extremely generous. He told me that they really wanted me back at my job and they didn't want to lose me; this filled me with confidence and I felt truly valued. He asked me to consider an offer of payment of half my salary but, as no one knew how long we would be in lock-down, they would review this on a month-by-month basis. I was incredibly grateful for this gesture as they were not obliged to pay me anything. I gratefully accepted their offer and thanked him for their generosity.

Chapter Twenty-One – Beyond My Limit

Throughout our house move, I had continued on my fitness journey with wonderful support from my trainer Bruno, but I had new goals! I had lost weight and now I wanted to build some muscle. I knew that all men's bodies were different and that's what makes us all unique but, to me, masculinity was about a well-toned and muscular body. I didn't want to look like one of the guys who take part in body-building competitions, I just wanted to shape my physique so that I could have a body I would be proud to show off.

We made plans to change my training programme to target specific areas of my body; this would involve less cardiovascular work and more weight lifting. The use of specific weights would target certain muscle groups and would enable me to build lean muscle. Bruno also changed my nutrition goals as I no longer needed to lose weight.

He told me that when he began training, he was like me. Both of us were over 30 and were struggling with a little excess baggage; I'm sure he won't mind me saying this as that's why he started out on his journey to fitness. He said that he felt out of place at the gym he was using as most of the people there were young and had amazing bodies. He had a PT there but he didn't get on with him, as he behaved like an army Sergeant Major. He decided to leave that gym to try to achieve his goals on his own. He began slowly, and found that the more he exercised and improved his knowledge of fitness and nutrition, the more he enjoyed it.

Over time, his fitness improved and he went on to do a number of challenges of physical strength and endurance; he wanted to experience pushing his body to its absolute limit. These challenges were completed in memory of his father, and to raise money for charity.

He told me that he had enjoyed his personal journey so much that he wanted to build his career around fitness, becoming the trainer that he would have wanted when he began his own journey. Listening to Bruno's story gave me all the inspiration I needed; if he could achieve his goals, there should be no reason for me not to be able to do something similar.

I decided to set myself an endurance challenge; I have never pushed myself beyond comfortable boundaries, and I felt that this was the right time for me to step out of my secure bubble. There was one person who had shown me how to do that – Bruno!

By now, we had been in lock-down for over two months, and the confinement that this brought with it definitely challenged me, both mentally and physically. As I have previously mentioned, I function well with focus and routine and, having these things stripped away by the lock-down, I found myself struggling; I needed to refocus and do something positive, not only for myself but, also, to help others.

I chose to do something that I knew would push me to my limit, not only physically, but also mentally. It was whilst

I was doing one of my regular work-outs on my cross trainer that I thought of the idea for my challenge. I decided that it was to be a five-hour continuous cross-trainer marathon and I would do this to raise money for Harrow Samaritans.

I had no idea if this was actually achievable, but I decided to do it anyway. When I began my fitness journey, I could barely do twenty minutes on the cross-trainer before I was exhausted but, during the time I was training to lose weight, I had managed to build that up to around one hour.

I set the date for the challenge; it would take place on May 30th 2020 and I thought that I would live-stream it so that friends and family could support me on the day.

I spoke to Bruno and he planned a training programme for me with the aim of increasing my endurance levels in preparation for the big day. I progressed well and felt focussed and structured again. Bruno told me that there would be some quite testing training sessions, but he said that he believed in me, and he had no doubt that I would smash the challenge. Hearing him say that he believed in me was probably one of the most amazing things he could have said. It gave my confidence a huge boost, and it certainly gave me the strength to get it done.

During the weeks leading to the challenge, my Mum called me to say that she had been asked whether she would be willing to be interviewed for the Harrow Samaritans Newsletter. One of the articles would be about my challenge and would ask why I had decided to support Harrow Samaritans. I told her that I had chosen the Harrow Branch of Samaritans for two reasons; the first being that the organisation provides invaluable support to those in crisis and that it is a vital resource. Unlike counsellors, Samaritan Volunteers provide support at a critical point in a person's life, as they are available twenty-four hours a day, seven days a week. My second reason for choosing them was because Mum is a volunteer at the Harrow Branch and she also became their Director for three years. She also helps with recruitment and training and, as do other Samaritan Volunteers, gives her time so selflessly.

Chapter Twenty-Two - Rising to the Challenge (pun intended!)

30th May 2020 - Challenge Day!.............

The plan for the day was to get up early, to prepare myself mentally for what lay ahead and also so that I could eat my training breakfast an hour before the start time. I was due to begin the challenge at 09:00 and complete it at 14:00. Carla was going to be my trusted assistant and it was her job to be in charge of all social media engagement.

Bruno had given me very specific instructions, and he said that would help me to get through the mental aspect of the challenge. He told me that I needed to break the five hours into individual hours to make the time more manageable. He said that if I planned to watch TV to keep me occupied, I would need to change what I was watching every hour so that I would begin each hour with something new and fresh; the reason for this was to create a specific mindset to allow me to cope with the whole challenge. He also said that doing the actual challenge would be very different to training for it as there would be a lot going on, plus adrenaline to push me through it.

I started my challenge on time and went live on Facebook so that our family and friends could see me begin. It was a very hot day and, although I had already decided that

I would do it in the coolest room in the house, it was still boiling!

We went live again about halfway through the challenge and again at the end. In between live 'broadcasts', Carla and I watched a film and some episodes of a series that we had been watching on Netflix. It was good to watch the TV as it allowed me to zone out. I was actually really surprised by how easy I was finding the challenge on the day - I was expecting to be really exhausted and also very bored. I think that there were lots of distractions that helped me through and, definitely, a sense of pride in what I was doing.

Throughout the live sections, I received a tremendous amount of support, not only from friends and family but, also, from the current Director of the Harrow Branch of the Samaritans for which I was raising the money. She commented a few times and said how wonderful I was and what this meant for her Branch and that she was extremely grateful. As with many businesses, charities were also suffering the effects of lock-down as many were relying on donations to keep going; the Samaritans Shop in Harrow was no different and needed to close temporarily. Before the challenge began, I had already raised almost £800, but the total rose as people donated throughout the five hours, so I knew that this was going to be a significant donation.

As I neared the end of the challenge, we went live for one final time so that everyone could see me finish. Again, there was a massive amount of support as we all did a final countdown. When I hit the five hours, I felt an enormous sense of relief, but also a sense of achievement- I was so proud of myself for getting it done.

I had never done anything like this before and I was amazed that I had actually completed it and not only that, the fund raised £1100. I was so grateful for all the support and donations from everybody and it made the whole thing totally worthwhile. Considering I set the fundraiser target at £100, I had smashed it. I had never believed that I would get anything near that amount and I would have been grateful for anything, so to hit this figure was absolutely brilliant.

Chapter Twenty Three – In My Forties and in Nappies

Although I have transitioned fully, I have been left with one issue that I feel I need to have resolved. As I mentioned earlier, I was having trouble with urine pooling in my urethra after urinating and this was still happening. Although this has been a problem since Stage Three, I didn't think anything could be done about it. I had seen posts on the surgery group from other guys who were also experiencing this issue, so it seemed to be a very common problem.

I had thought about contacting Mr Christopher to see if there was anything that he could do, surgically, to correct this. Although it doesn't cause me any pain or physical discomfort, it affects me psychologically as I have to wear a pad in my pants, like a nappy. I posted on the surgery group to ask for advice as to how I go about getting re-referred to Mr Christopher, and have been advised that all I need to do is to ask my GP to send a letter of referral to him.

I really don't relish the idea of having any more surgery, but I am hoping that it may be easily corrected and wouldn't involve anything too invasive. I would also want to have anything surgical carried out using a spinal block (an injection given in the spine to numb everything below the injection site) rather than a general anaesthetic. I really don't want to go through any more anaesthesia unless it's really necessary.

I made contact with Mr Christopher in May 2020 to ask for his advice and waited for him to call me back. When we finally talked, he said that I would need to be referred by my GP and then he would arrange for me to have a telephone consultation, rather than an in-person appointment, because of the Covid-19 lock-down situation.

I am yet to ask my GP for this referral because I haven't made up my mind about whether I want to actually go through further surgery. I know that I have been through so much to get to where I am now and it would be a shame not to be completely happy with the outcome, but I am just not sure yet. I will take some time to decide where I go from here.

Chapter Twenty-Four – Life Post-Sausage (aesthetics, sexual function, general function and user friendliness)

This final chapter was born whilst I was being pummelled into oblivion during a session with my osteopath.

Over the course of 3-4 osteopathy sessions, I had developed quite a friendly relationship with my osteopath, and I told him that I had written a book all about my life and transition and that the book was nearing the point when it would be sent off for editing. We chatted openly about my surgeries and he was so interested, not only from a medical stand-point, but also from his own personal curiosity. From the very first session, he made me feel comfortable and so I had no problem telling him all about my journey and the intricacies of full surgical transformation.

During a discussion about my ability to orgasm, he asked me if I had written about life after transition from the perspective of sexual function. I told him that, although I had talked about my choices with regard to the type of surgeries I had undergone and the potential impacts on sexual function, I hadn't talked about life afterward.

He told me that, as a reader, he would want to know if my choices had made an impact on my sexual function. I agreed that this should be included and I thanked him for pointing it out as it is a very important aspect of life, post transition.

So, let's talk about 'life post sausage'!

Warning: The following paragraphs contain very frank talk of sexual function. I give my apologies to my family, friends and anyone who knows me. I am probably just as embarrassed writing this as you will be reading it, but I think it would be remiss of me to leave it out.

I admit that there are certain aspects of my sex life, post transition, that are not quite as I would wish them to be. Some may think - don't be greedy, you have been changed in every aspect from being female to being male, and I have some sympathy with this point of view. I am so grateful for everything that those amazing doctors and surgeons have done to make me feel as though my body belongs to me, but to be honest, I wish certain things were different.

This is my User Review:

Let's start with **aesthetics**:

I am generally content with the way my sausage looks, but I know that I would have been happier with an uncircumcised look. However, I don't think that this is actually possible at this stage as the surgical technique isn't available. I would have been happier with 2 cylinders connected to the pump, rather than just one, and I would have liked larger testicular implants, which would have the capacity to hang more freely, like those of a natal male. Having said all of this, a surgeon can only work with what the patient has and if there is not enough skin, only small implants are possible. If there is insufficient room inside the phallus, only one cylinder can be used. I have to accept that the surgeons did an amazing job with what they had and that these things are just minor aesthetic issues.

Now let's talk about **sexual function**. This is where things get a little embarrassing, but here goes.....

As I mentioned earlier in my story, there are many choices to be made regarding the sexual elements of transition. These choices are made harder because we don't know what the outcomes will be as there are so many variables. We have to make our choices and pray that they will be the right ones down the line as, unfortunately, most of them are irreversible.

Having already chosen to go down the phalloplasty route, I already knew that I was dicing with the fact that I may have little if any sexual feeling in my willy. My further choices were to bury my clitoris and close my vaginal hole. Those choices were not easy to make because I was not only considering the impact that they may have on me, but also on my wife Carla. I discussed this with Carla and asked her what her thoughts were. She very bluntly told me that the decision had to be mine and mine alone. She was not being harsh, she just wanted me to make my own decisions based on my own wants and needs.

I chose to bury my clitoris for aesthetic reasons really as I thought it would look rather odd to have a mini willy underneath the phalloplasty. I suppose it would only be me and Carla that would see this, but I would know it was there and would worry that it would be noticeable at a urinal. I know, I know…. I can hear you saying it "who is going to be looking at a urinal" but these are the things we Trans people worry about.

I was told by my surgeon that I would still be able to access the clitoris after the burial, but that it would just be a little more difficult to stimulate because of its location.

Closing the vaginal hole was an easier decision for me as I just couldn't ever imagine leaving that open, it would just be odd. Plenty of people choose to leave it open and also the clitoris unburied because sexual function trumps aesthetics for them and their dysphoria may allow them to leave some of the female anatomy behind.

I have no regrets about closing my vaginal hole, but I do have some about burying my clitoris. Both Carla and I struggle with this aspect of my genitalia not being so accessible and this means that sex has changed significantly for us post-surgery. She struggles to do the right thing to stimulate it because of where it is. It is difficult, even for me, so I can only imagine the difficulty for her. What this means is that we have taken on different roles and although she can do other things to me, I have to bring myself to orgasm (cringing as I write!). It can, sometimes, take a very long time, as I now have to do things differently and then I feel under pressure to orgasm. Unfortunately, I am also unable to orgasm during penetration as, although I have some sexual sensation in my willy, it is more tactile sensation and this can be quite limiting.

We have talked openly about this and have come to the conclusion that I might just need to take the pressure off of myself and, if it happens, it happens, and if it doesn't, it doesn't. One of the many great things about my relationship with Carla is our ability to talk about things and I feel that we can move on from this and learn new ways of being together.

So, I suppose what I am saying is, with hindsight, I may have chosen differently, but how was I to know at the time?

As I have mentioned previously, I belong to some Trans groups online, one of them being a surgery phalloplasty group. There is not much information about phalloplasty surgery from people that have been through it, so this group is extremely valuable.

This group was my 'go to' place for any questions I had, from surgery preparation, to results, to healing etc. Occasionally, I still visit the site, even post-transition, as I like to keep up to date with new techniques and people's stories. I still get a little jealous when I hear other Trans guys talking about their results and the fact that they have great sexual function and sensation and the ability to orgasm easily but I have to accept that everyone heals differently, as the nerves that have to heal and grow after the surgeries, do so differently for everyone.

Lastly, I want to talk about **'user friendliness'**. I think it is important to talk about how easy it is to use my new appendage, as I know that when I was deciding which surgical route to take, this was one of my concerns.

I am extremely happy to report that it couldn't be easier to use as it is simply a matter of squeezing my right testicle a few times (like a pump) in the correct place. This allows the saline to travel from the reservoir in my abdomen and down the tube into the cylinder, giving the desired outcome (a boner). When finished, it is just as simple and involves squeezing quite hard on my right testicle and holding the squeeze to allow the saline to travel back up into the reservoir in my abdomen, giving the desired outcome (Mr Floppy).

My concern, pre-surgery, was that this process would detract from the sexual encounter. However, I would say that it is probably less of a distraction than putting on a condom, as other things can be done to distract from this. Carla has tried to use the pump, but we learned very quickly that if she slips, it can be incredibly painful.

One thing that I am 'over the moon' about, is being able to stand and pee at a urinal; I have a great aim! I will never understand how men manage to miss urinals/toilets and pee all over the floor when they were born with their equipment intact; I have only had my sausage for around 4 years, and this has never been a problem.

FYI and I have probably mentioned this earlier in the book: men's public toilets stink, but I am still overjoyed to be able to use them.

Overall, I am really happy with the outcomes of my surgeries, however, if I had known then what I know now, I may have chosen differently. Not knowing how things will turn out until after becoming fully healed is a problem. Advice is available but this is other people's perspectives, experiences and outcomes.

I don't want to put anyone off going through transition as this is my story and these are my results and, as I have said, everyone is different and will have different results.

I am just so happy to have been given the opportunity in my lifetime, to look in the mirror and to be able to see the real me.

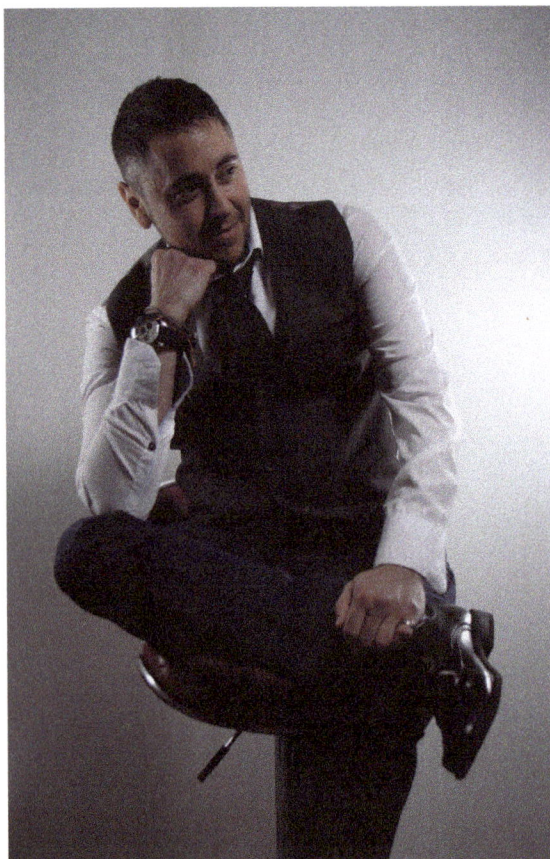

suited and booted

FINAL THOUGHTS

I am still reaching for my goals but, for once in my life, when I look in the mirror, I actually like what I see. I am not finished with my transformation by any means, but I am so happy with where I am right now.

I am so comfortable in my new body and it feels as if I was actually born this way; I don't regret a single moment of what I went through to get to this point. I am finally the man I should always have been. I am grateful to every single person who has been on my journey with me, Mum and Dad, Carla, my wonderful friends and extended family who have supported me without hesitation and without judgement, the doctors, nurses and surgeons who have helped me physically and psychologically to be the man I am today. Without all of these truly amazing people, I would have struggled and for that I am, and shall be, eternally grateful.

I finally found my 'happy ever after' with Carla and, considering I never thought I would find someone who wanted to be with me, let alone spend the rest of their life with me, I feel truly blessed!

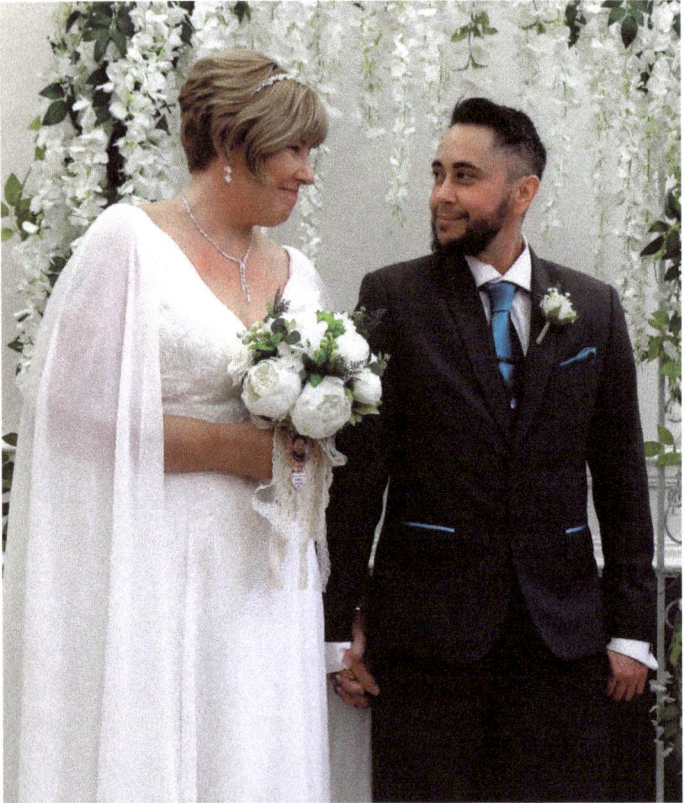

Wedding Photo

I don't ever want to forget my past; I am proud of where I have come from and the journey that I have taken to get to where I am today. It has been a physical and emotional roller-coaster in ways you cannot even imagine but, I am here, I am present and I am me!

My name is Daniel Kye Canter and I am still a work in progress....

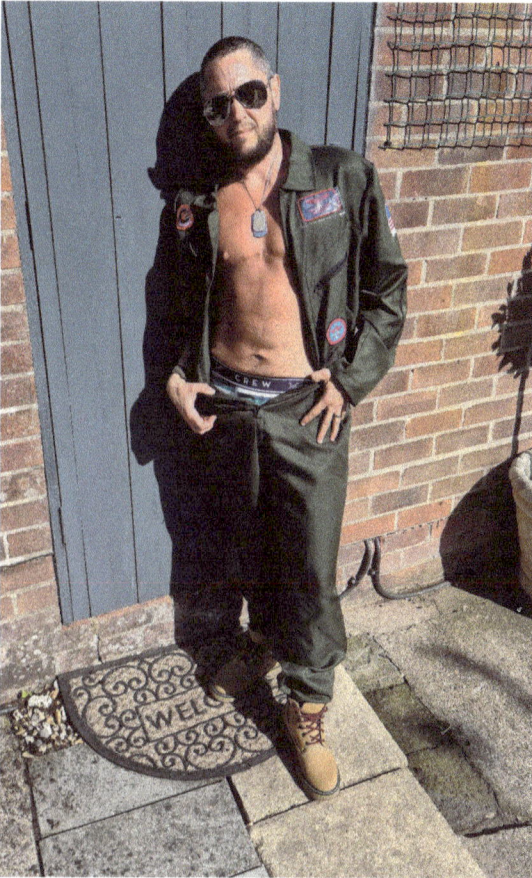

CPSIA information can be obtained
at www.ICGtesting.com
Printed in the USA
LVHW070343151021
700455LV00004B/4

9 781839 756115